FEDERALISM AND DECENTRALIZATION IN HEALTH CARE

A Decision Space Approach

Edited by Gregory P. Marchildon and Thomas J. Bossert

While health system decentralization is often associated with federations, there has been limited study on the connection between federalism and the organization of publicly financed or mandated health services. *Federalism and Decentralization in Health Care* discusses eight federations that differ in terms of their geography, history, and constitutional and political development. Looking at Canada, Brazil, Germany, Mexico, Nigeria, Pakistan, South Africa, and Switzerland, this volume examines constitutional responsibility for health care, the national laws establishing a right to health care, the predominant sources and organization of public revenues directed to health care, and the overall organization of the health system.

In additional to these structural features, each country case study is subjected to a "decision space analysis" to determine the actual degree of health system decentralization. This involves determining whether national and subnational governments have narrow, moderate, or broad discretion in their decisions on health system governance, access, human resources, organization, and financing. This comparative approach highlights similarities and differences among these federations. Offering reflections on recent trends in centralization or decentralization for the health system as a whole, *Federalism and Decentralization in Health Care* is a valuable resource for those studying health care policy in federal systems and especially those interested in comparative aspects of the topic.

GREGORY P. MARCHILDON is a professor and Ontario Research Chair in Health Policy and System Design in the Institute of Health Policy, Management and Evaluation at the University of Toronto.

THOMAS J. BOSSERT is a senior lecturer and the Director of the International Health Systems Program of the Harvard T.H. Chan School of Public Health.

Federalism and Decentralization in Health Care

A Decision Space Approach

EDITED BY GREGORY P. MARCHILDON
AND THOMAS J. BOSSERT

UNIVERSITY OF TORONTO PRESS
Toronto Buffalo London

© Forum of Federations 2018
Published by University of Toronto Press
Toronto Buffalo London
utorontopress.com
Printed and bound by CPI Group (UK) Ltd, Croydon, CR0 4YY

ISBN 978-1-4875-0159-4 (cloth)   ISBN 978-1-4875-2154-7 (paper)

Printed on acid-free, 100% post-consumer recycled paper with
vegetable-based inks.

Library and Archives Canada Cataloguing in Publication

Federalism and decentralization in health care : a decision space approach / edited by
Gregory P. Marchildon and Thomas J. Bossert.

Includes bibliographical references and index.
ISBN 978-1-4875-0159-4 (hardcover). – ISBN 978-1-4875-2154-7 (softcover)

1. Public health administration – Decentralization. 2. Medical policy. 3. Health
services administration. 4. Health planning. 5. Decentralization in government.
I. Marchildon, Gregory P., 1956–, editor II. Bossert, Thomas J., editor

RA393.F43 2018   362.1   C2017-906812-1

The Forum of Federations, the global network on federalism, supports better
governance through learning among federal experts and practitioners. Active on six
continents and supported by ten federal countries, it manages programs in established and emerging federations and publishes scholarly and educational materials.

University of Toronto Press acknowledges the financial assistance to its publishing
program of the Canada Council for the Arts and the Ontario Arts Council, an
agency of the Government of Ontario.

Canada Council   Conseil des Arts
for the Arts   du Canada

ONTARIO ARTS COUNCIL
CONSEIL DES ARTS DE L'ONTARIO
an Ontario government agency
un organisme du gouvernement de l'Ontario

Funded by the   Financé par le
Government   gouvernement
of Canada   du Canada

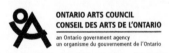

Contents

Tables, Figures, and Boxes

Tables

Figures

Boxes

A Note from the Forum of Federations

The current volume *Federalism and Decentralization in Health Care: A Decision Space Approach* is part of the Forum of Federations' ongoing commitment to shaping comparative research on federalism. It follows the Forum's work on structural issues of federalism published as a seven-volume set as part of the Global Dialogue Program, as well multi-country studies on capital cities, oil and gas, internal trade, metropolitan regions, political parties, intergovernmental relations, and, most recently, courts and judicial systems in federal countries. A forthcoming volume with the University of Toronto Press will cover public security.

Since the founding of the Forum of Federations, the issue of health care has been a core concern of its partners. Since 2001, a series of comparative projects have examined issues around the division of responsibilities, funding mechanisms, and means of cooperation between levels of government to ensure equity, access, quality, and efficiency of health care in federal systems. The objectives of the program have been to deepen knowledge on the issue and to draw out lessons for emerging federations. These projects have at different times responded to needs and requirements laid out by partners in Canada, Switzerland or Germany, Spain, Mexico, Brazil, India, Nigeria, and South Africa.

In classical federations, which were products of the nineteenth century, the lesser issues of education and health care were typically assigned to state or provincial governments. In time, however, provincial and national expenditures in these areas in OECD countries have taken on great fiscal and political importance. Thus policymakers must balance the needs and expectations of citizens, the demands of health care professionals, and the pressures on public budgets, and everywhere the trade-offs are becoming more difficult. In federal countries, these challenges are met through political institutions that require the participation and cooperation of two levels of government in the design and redesign of health policy, adding another layer of complexity to the management of health policies. This book makes a unique contribution to the study of public policy in the field of comparative federalism, decentralization, and health care policy. The countries examined in this volume are recognized as constitutional federations but differ in terms of the age, stability, and degree of decentralization within their respective federations. The economic and social circumstances of these countries also vary considerably. The countries can be classified into three groups: high-income (Switzerland, Canada, and Germany), high-middle-income (Brazil, Mexico, and South Africa) and low-middle-income (Nigeria and Pakistan).

Each chapter is written according to a template that allows for comparability and provides an overview of the federal structure, funding, and administration of the health system in a particular country, but goes beyond the constitutional assignment of roles and responsibilities to focus on the "decision space" that constituent units exercise in practice.

I am grateful to the individual authors for their contributions which add to the richness of this volume. I would also like to thank the editors, Gregory P. Marchildon and Thomas J. Bossert, for their skilled creation of this important work. They worked with us to conceptualize the project, shape the template, and edit this vast piece of research. I would like to thank my colleagues at the Forum, David Parks and Philip Gonzalez, for managing this project from start to finish, and John Light, for overseeing the publication process. Finally, thanks are due to our publisher, the University of Toronto Press, for their tireless work on this important volume.

Rupak Chattopadhyay
President and CEO, Forum of Federations

Acknowledgments

We would like to thank the Forum of Federations, an international network of federal countries that was initially established by the Government of Canada, for sponsoring this research. We are particularly indebted to Rupak Chattopadhyay, the president of the Forum, and to his staff and consultants, especially David Parks, who was heavily involved in the early stages of the project. We are grateful for the support of the Canada Research Chair and the Ontario Research Chair programs and the International Health Systems Program in the Department of Global Health and Population at the Harvard T.H. Chan School of Public Health. We thank Alex Titeu at the University of Toronto's Institute of Health Policy, Management, and Evaluation for his technical support on the final manuscript. We very much appreciated the University of Toronto Press and its extensive review and editorial process for making this a better book. We sincerely thank our editor, Stephen Shapiro, for his enthusiastic support of this project and book. Finally, we would like to thank our chapter contributors, who stuck with us on this very long journey from our workshop in Boston in 2012 to publication.

FEDERALISM AND DECENTRALIZATION IN HEALTH CARE

Chapter One

An Introduction to Federalism and Decentralization in Health Care

GREGORY P. MARCHILDON AND THOMAS J. BOSSERT

Introduction

Federalism and decentralization are related concepts that have engaged social scientists and practitioners in theoretical and empirical debates for generations, as summarized by Banting and Corbett (2002) and Costa-Font and Greer (2013). They are related in the sense that federalism by definition involves a degree of political, fiscal, and administrative decentralization, while the broader term "decentralization" deals with contexts well beyond federalism (Bankauskaite & Saltman, 2007). Unfortunately, there is little consensus among scholars and decision makers about how these two terms should be defined, how they are related, what categories are useful to analyse them, and what impact they have on the social objectives we might want to achieve (Adolph, Greer, & Massard da Fonseca, 2012). These concepts are more than an academic problem as they currently engage policymakers in many countries who are coping with how to design their health systems to be both more effective and more responsive to their populations. Federalism and decentralization appear on the policy agenda in many countries repeatedly.

This volume focuses on health care, one of the most financially onerous and contested social policy responsibilities of governments in the early twenty-first century. This alone might be sufficient justification for a study of the nexus between federalism and decentralization (and its converse, centralization). However, it needs to be emphasized that decentralization is a relative concept that can only be understood given a particular historical and comparative context. Is the health system of a given federation decentralizing or centralizing relative to its past? And is the health system of a given federation decentralized or centralized relative to the federations to which it is being compared? For the purposes of this study, we defined federalism as a multi-tiered government combining elements of shared-rule and regional self-rule where constituent unit autonomy is generally guaranteed by a constitution regarded as the highest law of the land (Marchildon, 2013).

The sponsor of this project is the Forum of Federations, a global network on federalism and multilevel government that supports better governance through learning among both practitioners and experts, including scholars. Established in the late 1990s with a sizeable seed investment from the Government of Canada, the Forum is active on six continents, running programs in over twenty countries that range from long-established federations to those countries transitioning from highly centralized forms of governance to decentralized structures. While the Forum has examined numerous policy domains since its creation in the late 1990s, this is the first project to address the relationship between federalism and health system decentralization involving countries that vary considerably in terms of economic development, wealth disparities, average income, administrative capacity, and political evolution.

In the summer of 2011, we were asked by the Forum to conduct a multi-country study on this subject in response to the interest of some of the Forum's member countries. The eight case studies of countries included in this volume reflect the interests of those members who had a deep concern with this particular subject at the time they were asked. This "coalition of the willing" may seem a highly opportunistic method of country selection. However, those Forum members with an interest in the project also represented countries in which federalism and decentralization in the governance, financing, administration, or delivery of health care is perceived to be a major challenge. In addition, the majority of the health systems in these nations, with the exception of the highest-income countries, are deeply understudied. This particular selection of case studies also offered a good range of different approaches to federalism and health system decentralization upon which to draw policy lessons and, for those understudied countries, a base line for future scholarly investigation.

With the assistance of the Forum, we selected a lead author for each of the countries. At a workshop held at the Harvard T.H. Chan School of Public Health (then the Harvard School of Public Health) in Boston in March 2012, these lead authors presented a concise summary of their study based on a framework of common questions developed months before. For this workshop, we attempted to introduce rigour into the comparative study by developing a detailed, common template for the authors, who were then asked to refine their drafts based on the feedback received at the workshop. This template was based on a comparative policy methodology developed by Rose (2005) and the use of decision space analysis as originally proposed by Bossert (1998) and as subsequently developed and used in the health systems literature (Roman, Cleary, & McIntyre, 2017). Whereas most conceptual frameworks on decentralization tend to privilege structure, decision space analysis evaluates the implementation and ongoing management – the practices on the ground of any health system. We therefore used decision space analysis as the conceptual framework in organizing comparisons of the eight health system studies in this book.

Every health system is made up of policy program elements. The key conceptual task according to Rose (2005) is to identify the common elements or categories that can be usefully compared across jurisdictions. For this particular study, we asked authors to identify and describe five structural features in each federation based on our past experience in conducting comparative health systems studies: 1) the assignment of constitutional responsibility for health and health care within the federation; 2) the existence (or not) of a national law on health care establishing rights and responsibilities; 3) the predominant sources of revenue directed to public-sector health care and the public and private sources and proportion of financing; 4) the funding and budgeting process of the central government's health ministry relative to the funding and budgeting processes for the subnational governments; and 5) the organization of the publicly financed or subsidized part of the health system.

Using the decision space analysis approach, we then required each author to address the following issues related to health system decentralization:

- the range of decision space choices (narrow, moderate, broad) in terms of governance rules, access rules, health human resources, health organization, and financing;
- the capacities of subnational governments and delegated health authorities at the subnational level;
- the relative reliance of subnational governments on external (central government revenues) as opposed to internal revenues for health expenditures;
- the extent of conditionality attached to central government health transfers to subnational governments;
- the nature of the interactions between central and subnational governments in terms of health policy and planning, including the intergovernmental mechanisms;
- the trends in the last five to ten years in terms of health system decentralization or centralization.

Based upon the discussion in the workshop, we produced a working glossary involving a few key terms used in the dual literatures of federalism and health system decentralization. The case study chapters underwent two further rounds of editorial feedback and redrafting before going through peer review and a final draft.

With the exception of Pakistan, which was subsequently selected by the editors as a case study as a consequence of its recent experiment in radical decentralization, the countries examined in this volume were self-selected by the members of the Forum of Federations. However, the template and glossary ensured that similar questions were being asked in all cases so that we could reap at least two of the benefits of comparative policy analysis. In particular, we wanted to "provide learning opportunities" to decision makers and scholars from these diverse policy experiences (Marmor, Freeman, & Okma, 2005, p. 335). Given the nature of the cases and what we think is the danger of inferring causal links between the structure of a particular federation and its health system, we did not design the study as a series of "quasi-natural" experiments (Marmor et al., 2005, p. 336) where we would be able to point to recent changes to health decentralization as causing differences in health system performance or health outcomes. There are simply too many confounding variables to allow for this. Moreover, the time between reform and the impact this might have is often too short. Finally, we felt that a more nuanced and qualitative assessment through a decision space analysis would prove more useful than trying to link health system outcomes to shifts along the continuum of centralization and decentralization, even if this approach might not generate definitive conclusions.

The countries in all eight case studies share one feature in common – they are recognized as constitutional federations (Griffiths, 2002). At the same time, they differ in terms of the age, stability, and degree of political, fiscal, and constitutional decentralization. Moreover, each of these federations had a unique historical evolution. This collection of eight case studies on federalism and the health sector shows that, far from being simple categories, federalism and health system decentralization involve complex administrative and political structures, with considerable variation. The economic and social circumstances of these countries also vary considerably. For example, as measured by gross national income per capita (US$ – purchase power parity), the average incomes in the countries ranged from a high of $82,730 (Switzerland) to a low of $1,260 (Pakistan) in 2012. Based on the World Bank rankings, the countries can be classified into three groups: high-income (Canada, Germany, and Switzerland), high-middle-income (Brazil, Mexico, and South Africa), and low-middle-income (Nigeria and Pakistan).

When conducting comparative policy research, history and context matter (Ashfort, 1992; Fierlbeck & Palley, 2015; Maioni, 1998; Tuohy, 1999). While some of the federations in this study have experienced long periods of peace and great political stability, others have suffered through protracted periods of war and dictatorship. Indeed, some countries face ongoing threats of secession from some of their constituent units and the possibility of civil war, factors that can have a pronounced impact on the structure and management of these federations (Marchildon, 2009). These differing contexts must be appreciated in any discussion of common trends in terms of health system structures, including tendencies to move to greater centralization or decentralization.

In some ways, this study could be viewed as a subset of studies of health system decentralization (e.g., Saltman, Bankauskaite, & Vrangbæk, 2007) that focus on the constitutional assignment of health system responsibilities and fiscal capacities to specific governmental levels. Alternatively, decentralization could be perceived as the actual roles and responsibilities exercised by each level of government within a federation, whether or not assigned by a constitution. We have combined both approaches in this book, and the results are summarized in the concluding chapter.

Constitutions, Federalism, and Decentralization

As the supreme written law of a country, a constitution is not amendable except through a procedure that generally requires the consent of a significant proportion of the constituent units. These constituent units – known as states, provinces, cantons, or *Länder* depending on the country – are orders of government with a parallel authority to that of the central government with the ability to act directly for their respective residents. Although the phrase "orders of government" is used in some countries to define the relationship between constitutionally recognized governments, in other countries, the term "levels of government" is more commonly used, and the two terms are treated as the same for the purposes of this book.

In all cases, constitutions assign powers to the central government and the constituent units. As will be seen, in some countries, powers are constitutionally divided between two levels of government, and in other countries, among three levels of government – that is, among central, regional, and local governments. There is nothing new in the multilevel governance of health care, but with constitutional federations, the starting point for understanding how a particular health system is configured begins with an examination of the country's constitution.

Constitutions in some countries assign powers in health and health care to respective orders of government in watertight compartments. In contrast, other countries have constitutions which ignore health care as a category, and responsibility and authority must be inferred from more general language. In a few cases, constitutions assign the responsibility for health care to two or more levels of government in "concurrent" lists of functions that are either shared or managed in a parallel fashion. In these last cases, it is essential to examine the actual practices of the governments that constitute a federation to determine the degree of health system centralization or decentralization.

In some instances, the fiscal capacity of the constituent unit is sufficient to carry out its health system responsibilities, but in others the constituent unit is almost entirely reliant on fiscal transfers from the central government and thus subject to considerable political pressure and influence in the exercise of its authority. Sometimes, a central government establishes a right of access to health care that may create an obligation that the constituent units only have limited capacity to deliver – what some might call an unfunded or underfunded mandate.

Examination of any health system centralization or decentralization in federal countries must be put into the context of the overall decentralization of these particular federations. In the federalism literature, two ways have been devised to measure the degree of decentralization. The first method is to determine the fiscal capacity of the central government relative to the constituent units within a given federation. This analysis was completed by federalism scholar Ron Watts for all the case studies included in this volume except Pakistan (Watts, 2008).

Table 1.1 presents the countries in this study ranked in ascending order of the central governments' revenues (before transfers) as a percentage of total government revenues. The first column illustrates the federal government's fiscal capacity, including its potential to use transfers to subnational governments to exercise its policy influence – generally referred to as the spending power in federal systems (Watts, 2009). It is interesting to note that the higher the average per capita income in a country, the greater the degree of decentralization, whereas lower per capita incomes are associated with more centralized federations.

The second column in Table 1.1 provides an overall picture of the degree to which constituent units within federations are reliant on central government revenues. Health care can be one of the most extensive areas of responsibility assumed by constituent units within federations, and the revenues needed to deliver these services come from some combination of own-source revenues and transfers from the central government. The third column in Table 1.1 presents the expenditures of central governments as a percentage of all government (federal, regional, local) spending once all transfers have been made.

While Table 1.1 provides a snapshot of the fiscal resources actually held by constituent units in the exercise of the responsibilities, it does not tell us very much about the political and constitutional factors that shape the way a federation actually operates. These latter factors have been captured in an index produced by Requejo (2010), who has compared federations based on their respective degree of both de facto decentralization and constitutional decentralization. The former is calculated on a host of political and fiscal factors and

Table 1.1 Fiscal capacity of central governments relative to constituent units, 2000–4

Federal country case studies	Central government revenues (before transfers) as a % of total government revenues	Central government transfers as a % of constituent unit revenues	Central government expenditures (after transfers) as a % of total government expenditures
Switzerland	40.0	24.8	32.0
Canada	47.2	12.9	37.0
Germany	65.0	43.8	37.0
Brazil	69.2	30.0	59.5
South Africa	82.0	96.1	50.0
Mexico	91.3	87.9	58.7
Nigeria	98.0	89.0	59.7

Source: Derived from Watts (2008), Table 9 (p. 102), Table 10 (p. 103), and Table 11 (p. 105).

Table 1.2 Degree of actual and constitutional decentralization based on 20-point scale

Federal country case studies	Degree of de facto federalism	Degree of structural decentralization
Canada	16.5	13.0
Switzerland	14.0	15.0
Germany	12.0	14.0
Brazil	11.0	13.5
South Africa	7.0	9.0
Mexico	5.0	11.0

Source: Derived from Requejo (2010, p. 287), Table 13.2.

outcomes, while the latter is based on the constitutional division of powers and formal governmental structures. Each of these forms of decentralization is enumerated on a 20-point scale (with 20 being the most decentralized) based on a broad range of indicators including, for example, the constitutional guarantee of subnational self-government; an upper chamber with representatives appointed by subnational institutions; the assignment of unallocated powers to subnational governments; and the regulated right of secession of at least some subnational units (Requejo, 2010). Table 1.2 summarizes Requejo's results for six of our country case studies (Pakistan and Nigeria were not assessed in his study).

The results are mainly consistent with Table 1.1, with two important differences. First, Canada is more decentralized than its constitutional form would imply, a result that is consistent with the high degree of fiscal autonomy exercised by provincial governments in that country. Second, South Africa is less decentralized than its formal governmental structure would indicate, a fact also consistent with the fiscal power of the central government and the correspondingly limited fiscal capacity of provincial governments in that country.

In the last decade, a group of scholars has developed a more sophisticated comparative measurement of the power and authority of sub-federal states, what they call regional governments, which are located between the national and local levels of government (Hooghe et al., 2016; Marks, Hooghe, & Schakel, 2008). The regional authority instrument (RAI) created by this group involves indicators of the extent to which subnational states are capable of self-rule and the extent to which they participate in national policy and government (shared-rule). As a result, RAI is not a straightforward indicator of decentralization, and in fact, due in part to the *Länder*'s significant involvement in national-level decision-making, Germany receives a much higher RAI score than countries which are considerably more decentralized, such as Switzerland and Canada. In addition, data has not yet been established for three of the countries covered in this study: South Africa, Brazil, and Nigeria (Hooghe et al., 2016).

The analysis in this section focused on the general characteristics of a country's federalism and decentralization; next we look specifically at these characteristics of the health system.

Health System Decentralization in Practice and the Decision Space Framework

To provide a comparative framework for this study, we examined health system decentralization in terms of the "decision space" that constituent units exercise in practice. This allowed us to get beyond the constitutional assignment of roles and responsibilities for specific health functions, policies, and programs to the other laws and intergovernmental practices that determine the actual autonomy of constituent units relative to the central government. This analysis was first developed, applied, and extended by one of the editors in earlier works (Bossert, 1998; Bossert, 2015; Mitchell & Bossert, 2010). This decision space is categorized according to the degree of decision-making choice in terms of key functions, shown in Table 1.3, and subfunctions under each function.

The *financing* functions focused on how much choice the subnational units had for raising revenue and allocating expenditures. If the central government provides most of the revenue through intergovernmental transfers, then the decision space was deemed to be *narrow*; if funding mainly came from sources internal to the subnational unit, then it would be *wide*; and if there was a balanced mix or if the intergovernmental transfers were not limited by conditions, it would be considered *moderate*.

Table 1.3 Health care decision space for subnational states within federations

Functions	Range of Choice		
	Narrow	Moderate	Wide
Financing (revenue and expenditures)	Central funding	Mixed funding	Local funding
Service organization and delivery (required programs, payment mechanisms, autonomy of hospitals, and local insurance plans)	Central definitions and requirements	Some range of local choice	Few limits on local choice
Human resources (salaries, contracting, civil service rules)	Central definitions and requirements	Some range of local choice	Few limits on local choice
Access rules (targeting, benefits)	Central definitions and requirements	Some range of local choice	Few limits on local choice
Governance rules (accountability and governance structures)	Central definitions and requirements	Some range of local choice	Few limits on local choice

Source: Derived from Bossert (1998) and Mitchell and Bossert (2010)

Similarly for expenditures, if budget expenditures at subnational units had to be approved by the national level, then the decision space would be *narrow*. Expenditure decision space would be *wide* if there were few restrictions, and if subnational choice was allowed but had some restrictions it was *moderate*.

Service organization includes autonomous hospitals, local insurance plans, payment mechanisms, and norms and standards including required programs. Again, if subnational units had little choice in these areas, the decision space was deemed to be *narrow*. If it was without much restriction from the national level, decision space was *wide*, and if there was a range of choices but within limits set by central restrictions, it was *moderate*. In many countries national control over norms, standards, and required programs is a significant means by which central authorities restrict local choice.

Human resources is a major area of decision-making and one often defined by national rules. Choices over salary levels, making contracts with individual providers, and civil service rules are *narrow* if the central authorities control these human resources functions. They are *wide* if subnational units can make most of these choices and *moderate* if there is some choice but clear restrictions imposed by the national government.

Access rules define the populations that are targeted for specific attention, especially for subsidies, free access to public facilities, or social insurance. If the national government or the constitution defines this population (for instance, a "right to health" provision that is enforced) then the local choice is *narrow*. If subnational units are able to define priorities to different populations, then the choice is *wide*, and if there is a mix of choice, it is *moderate*.

Governance rules involve choices of the composition of facility boards, district offices, and types of community participation. Again, the local choice is *narrow* if these subfunctions are defined by national rules or practice, *wide* if local authorities can make most of the choices, and *moderate* if there is some choice but it is limited by national rules.

The authors were faced with many judgment calls for these general categories. However, the drafts were reviewed by the editors to try to make the comparisons of the decision space for these functions consistent among the countries.

We then asked authors to focus on three areas associated with health system decentralization. The first was capacity, specifically the fiscal capacity of constituent units to generate their own-source revenues and the administrative (i.e., human) capacity to regulate, implement, and manage subnational health systems. The second was central government fiscal transfers to constituent units, describing the proportion and extent to which health transfers are conditional or unconditional, the extent to which the transferring government achieves its policy purpose (if possible), and the extent of policy autonomy of receiving governments. Finally, our authors were asked to describe the intergovernmental processes and agencies as well as the coordinating mechanisms with some assessment of the federalism culture as they pertain to health care policies and programs.

In the final section, authors describe what they perceived to be the recent trends in centralization or decentralizations for the health system as a whole. Although we recognize that this portion of the discussion is somewhat speculative, it is grounded in a careful study of the existing constitutional distribution of powers as well as the actual decision space choices exercised by subnational states within each country. This kind of informed speculation is essential to understanding the influence of federalism on health system policy-setting and decision-making.

Given the very different histories and contexts of the federations in this study, the authors needed considerable latitude in selecting the key functions and subfunctions relevant to their respective case studies. Moreover, they had to exercise considerable judgment in deciding the degree of functional decision-making exercised by subnational states. In the concluding chapter, we use the analyses and judgments in the eight case studies to draw some conclusions concerning the overall degree of health system decentralization and where these countries sit in relation to each other. Based on the results, we were also able to make some policy recommendations to decision makers considering decentralization structures and processes in their respective health systems in order to improve overall performance or implement a given set of reforms.

We present the country case studies in order of the three income categories as classified by the World Bank and the degree of decentralization we found in our decision space analysis. The high-income countries of Canada, Switzerland, and Germany make up the first group of case studies. Canada and Switzerland vie for the position of having the most decentralized health systems in the Organisation for Economic Co-operation and Development (OECD). In contrast, Germany has a comparatively centralized health system. The remaining high-middle- and low-middle-income countries are presented in order of the degree of health system decentralization, with the most extreme example of decentralization – Pakistan – going first, followed by South Africa, Brazil, Mexico, and finally Nigeria as the most centralized health system case study in this volume.

In the final chapter, we summarize our findings and draw some policy lessons. We were impressed by the extent to which formal constitutions can and do play a major role in shaping – as well as setting a boundary around – the health system decentralization. At the same time, lawmaking (whether through constitution or regular statute) can never assure effective health system decentralization. Successful health system decentralization depends on the governance, fiscal, administrative, and human resource capacities of subnational levels of government. The type and level of capacity required depend to some extent on the form of decentralization selected. For example, more market-based forms of decentralization require a high degree of regulatory capacity, while state-based forms of decentralization require a corps of effective public administrators and service deliverers. Because of the economies of scale and scope, it does seem that certain functions – such as immunization, epidemic control, drug control including pharmaceutical safety, and health facility and professional accreditation – are better exercised by the national government. However, it is possible to achieve national standards and policies without centralization if the appropriate intergovernmental institutions and processes are in place so that subnational governments can fill the role usually played by central governments acting alone.

REFERENCES

Adolph, C., Greer, S.L., & Massard da Fonseca, E. (2012). Allocation of authority in European health policy. *Social Science & Medicine, 75*(9), 1595–603. https://doi.org /10.1016/j.socscimed.2012.05.041

Ashfort, D.H. (Ed.). (1992). *History and context in comparative public policy.* Pittsburgh, PA: University of Pittsburgh Press.

Bankauskaite, V., & Saltman, R.B. (2007). Central issues in the decentralization debate. In R.B. Saltman, V. Bankauskaite, & K. Vrangbæk (Eds.), *Decentralization in health care* (pp. 9–21). Maidenhead, UK: Open University Press.

Banting, K.G., & Corbett, S.M. (Eds.). (2002). *Health policy and federalism: A comparative perspective on multi-level governance.* Montreal, QC: McGill-Queen's University Press.

Bossert, T.J. (1998). Analyzing the decentralization of health systems in developing countries: Decision space, innovation and performance. *Social Science & Medicine, 47*(10), 1513–27. https://doi.org/10.1016/S0277-9536(98)00234-2

Bossert T.J. (2015). Empirical studies of an approach to decentralization: "Decision space" in decentralized health systems. In J.-P. Faguet & C. Pöschl (Eds.), *Is decentralization good for development?: Perspectives from academics and policy makers* (pp. 277–298). London, UK: Oxford University Press.

Costa-Font, J., & Greer, S.L. (Eds.). (2013). *Federalism and decentralization in European health and social care.* Basingstoke, UK: Palgrave Macmillan. https://doi.org/10.1057/9781137291875

Fierlbeck, K., & Palley, H.A. (2015). Comparative policy analysis, health care, and federal systems. In K. Fierlbeck & H.A. Palley (Eds.), *Comparative health care federalism* (pp. 1–15). London, UK: Routledge.

Griffiths, A.L. (Ed.). (2002). *Handbook of federal countries, 2002.* Montreal, QC: McGill-Queen's University Press for the Forum of Federations.

Hooghe, L., Marks, G., Schakel, A.H., Osterkatz, S.C., Niedzwiecki, S., & Shair-Rosenfield, S. (2016). *Measuring regional authority: A postfunctionalist theory of governance* (Vol. 1). Oxford, UK: Oxford University Press. https://doi.org/10.1093/acprof:oso/9780198728870.001.0001

Maioni, A. (1998). *Parting at the crossroads: The emergence of health insurance in the United States and Canada.* Princeton, NJ: Princeton University Press.

Marchildon, G.P. (2009). Postmodern federalism and sub-state nationalism. In A. Ward & L. Ward (Eds.), *The Ashgate research companion to federalism* (pp. 441–55). Farnham, UK: Ashgate.

Marchildon, G.P. (2013). The future of the federal role in Canadian health care. In K. Fierlbeck & W. Lahey (Eds.), *Health care federalism in Canada: Critical junctures and critical perspectives* (pp. 177–91). Montreal, QC: McGill-Queen's University Press.

Marks, G., Hooghe, L., & Schakel, A.H. (2008). Measuring regional authority. *Regional & Federal Studies, 18*(2–3), 111–21. https://doi.org/10.1080/13597560801979464

Marmor, T., Freeman, R., & Okma, K. (2005). Comparative perspectives and policy learning in the world of health care. *Journal of Comparative Policy Analysis, 7*(4), 331–48. https://doi.org/10.1080/13876980500319253

Mitchell, A., & Bossert, T.J. (2010). Decentralization, governance and health-system performance: "Where you stand depends on where you sit." *Development Policy Review, 28*(6), 669–91. https://doi.org/10.1111/j.1467-7679.2010.00504.x

Roman, T.E., Cleary, S., & McIntyre, D. (2017). Exploring the functioning of decision space: A review of the available health systems literature. *International Journal of Health Policy and Management, 6*(x), 1–12, online first. https://doi.org/10.15171/ijhpm.2017.26

Rose, R. (2005). *Learning from comparative public policy: A practical guide.* London, UK: Routledge.

Requejo, F. (2010). Federalism and democracy: The case of minority nations – a federalist deficit. In M. Burgess & A. Gagnon (Eds.), *Federal democracies* (pp. 275–98). London, UK: Routledge.

Saltman, R.B., Bankauskaite, V., & Vrangbæk, K. (Eds.). (2007). *Decentralization in health care.* Maidenhead, UK: McGraw Hill–Open University Press.

Tuohy, C.H. (1999). *Accidental logics: The dynamics of change in the health care arena in the United States, Britain, and Canada.* Oxford, UK: Oxford University Press.

Watts, R.L. (2008). *Comparing federal systems* (3rd ed.). Kingston, ON: McGill-Queen's University Press for the Institute of Intergovernmental Relations.

Watts, R.L. (2009). *The spending power in federal systems: A comparative study.* Kingston, ON: Institute of Intergovernmental Relations.

Chapter Two

Switzerland: Subnational Authority and Decentralized Health Care

BJÖRN UHLMANN

Structural Features of the Swiss Federation

Since the beginning of the modern Swiss constitution in 1848, federalism served as a political device to peacefully accommodate religious and linguistic minorities in the Swiss federation. Because the constitution was built upon the events of a civil war (Sonderbundskrieg) in 1847 fought between progressive urban Reformists, in favour of a strong centralized state, and conservative rural Catholics, who favoured a federation with highly autonomous cantons, the founding fathers thought it wise to tip the balance of political power between the centre (confederation) and the states (known as cantons) in favour of the cantons. They created political room for the self-determination of culturally diverse communities in a larger union. Consequently, the Swiss federation was composed of different member nations, each rather homogeneous within itself, but quite heterogeneous within the union, creating a "federation of nations" (Kriesi, 1999, p. 18). By its character, the constitution was more confederal – where member states remain the locus of sovereignty and retain the bulk of powers, assigning a minimum of legislative powers and responsibilities to a central government – than a federal constitution which aims at creating a balance between national and subnational governments (Hueglin & Fenna, 2005, pp. 34–5). While jurisdiction over the military, the national reserve, and currency was placed in the hands of the confederation, most other areas of jurisdiction – such as health, education, and religious, cultural, and linguistic affairs – remained with the cantons.

Although there has been an increase in federal legislative and executive power since 1848, the main characteristics of the Swiss federation remain the same. All twenty-six cantons possess their own constitution and own local governments and maintain separate judicial systems. Cantons are sovereign in legislative matters, and they do not delegate legislative power to federal authorities.

This means in particular that they can raise – as can the confederation and the municipalities – their own taxes and decide in what area they want to spend the funds. Cantonal taxation and allocation power is an important feature of Swiss federalism since it allows the cantons to stay – to a considerable degree – financially and politically independent of the federal authorities.

In contrast to the more centralized German federal system, for example, the Swiss federal system is highly decentralized (Braun, 2003). Although the Swiss federation does not show the same high degree of decentralization as Canada and is closer to the United States or Belgium in Requejo's cross-country comparison of decentralization (Requejo, 2006), it means nevertheless that Switzerland has not been able to achieve national standards in public policies across its cantonal borders, and this has allowed diverse, and to some extent unequal, social and health policies.

This chapter aims to give an overview of political institutions in Switzerland and their impact on health affairs. Based on this evidence, the Swiss health system is then gauged according to Bossert's concept of decision space (Bossert, 1998) in order to assess the range of cantonal power and resulting decentralization in the Swiss health system. Finally, the general trends in terms of health system decentralization are described.

Constitutional Design and Health Authority

In contrast to Australia and Canada, which are federal but majoritarian Westminster-style democracies based historically on a two-party system – one in government and another in opposition – Switzerland's democracy was founded on a multiparty system and a political culture of consensus (Lijphart, 1999). This culture of concordance (*Konkordanzsystem*) is shaped by its political institutions such as the confederal arrangements and popular rights (Linder & Steffen, 2007). Conflict resolution is achieved through negotiation and compromise, while politics generally takes place within a framework of consensus rather than competition.

The referendum plays an important role in consensus-oriented policymaking in Switzerland. According to the Federal Constitution of Switzerland,[1] 50,000 Swiss citizens or eight cantons can ask for a (facultative) referendum on federal laws. Referendums are only possible after the decision-making process in Parliament; however, the possibility of a referendum casts its shadow on deliberations in Parliament. In case of success, the referendum is a very

---

1 Article 141, Federal Constitution of Switzerland, 18 April 1999.

effective veto instrument, since the actor receives legitimation for his interests by the highest democratic institution: the electorate.[2] Popular initiatives and referendums[3] in health affairs occur quite often, and citizens and political parties use them actively to promote their interests (Immergut, 1990; Immergut, 1992; Uhlmann & Braun, 2011).

Regarding the federal structure, there are three layers of government recognized in the confederation's constitution, a structure that has multiple veto points and opportunities for actors at different administrative and political levels (Immergut, 1990; Immergut, 1992; Tsebelis, 2002). The first layer, the central government, is made up of the executive Federal Council (Bundesrat) and the legislative two-chamber Parliament. The Federal Council consists of seven members and is a collective body. Each member shares the same power and weight in the council. Each member of the Council is a principal of a public administration department, accountable for the execution of his or her department (e.g., defence, health, and social policy). Since there are only seven departments, the responsibility held by each member is much larger than those held by ministers and their respective ministries in most other countries. The bicameral Parliament elects the members of the Federal Council for fixed four-year terms. The Council or its members cannot be recalled.

Members of the Federal Council are elected based on party affiliation, with linguistic and regional origins taken into consideration in order to achieve a balanced representation. Cantonal governments have no input into the election of the Federal Council. The federal political system is a mixture between a presidential (fixed-term) system, a majoritarian system (where a majority of the federal Parliament elects the Council), and a French-style directorial (executive Council of Peers) system of government democracy. The seven members of the Federal Council elect, from their ranks, the president of the Swiss federation for a period of one year. The president has no additional political power other than to serve as a representative of the country.

The second layer of governmental order is the canton. All twenty-six cantons have a structure that parallels the federal political system: they possess directorial executive bodies and legislative cantonal parliaments based on a multiparty consensual system, as well as taxing and spending power and their own courts.

---

2 For an explanation of referendums in Switzerland and their effectiveness, see Kriesi (1998), Linder (2005), and Sciarini (2007); for a broader discussion of functions and dysfunctions of referendums, see Papadopoulos (1995).

3 For referendum examples in Swiss health affairs, see Immergut (1992) and Uhlmann and Braun (2011).

However, the cantonal executive bodies are elected not by Parliament but directly by the people of the respective cantons. As in the federal level of government, members of the cantonal executive bodies are the ministers of departments and directly accountable to the electorate for their administration.

On the federal level, cantons are represented in the "Council of the States," the Senate (Ständerat), of the bicameral Parliament. The political rights of the councillors (Ständerate) are the same as those of the House of Representatives (Nationalrat). However, the influence of the cantons in national lawmaking in the Council of the States is weak compared to the Länder in Germany. Since the councillors are elected directly by their cantonal electorate, they vote without cantonal instructions, making it harder for the cantonal executives to defend their interests in national lawmaking. This is especially important in policy areas such as health care, where the cantons have considerable legislative power.

The cantons hold residual legislative powers in that all powers that are not explicitly assigned to the federation are reserved for the cantons. However, they collectively have the power to delegate legislative powers to the confederation. Any transmission of such powers, including the authority to legislate on health insurance, hospitals, nursing, and medical practitioners, must be constitutionally authorized through the existing federal constitution or through a new amendment. Amendments need to be approved by both the majority of the cantons and the majority of the Swiss electorate, a process known as a double majority quorum.

Regarding health, several articles in the federal constitution provide the foundation for the confederation's legislative powers. However, the majority of these powers are concurrent or shared with the cantons. Furthermore, the federal constitution stipulates the basic principle that, first and foremost, individuals take responsibility for their own welfare and health care, and only on a subsidiary base should the state complement individual responsibility.[4] The same article states that the confederation and the cantons have to ensure that every person living in Switzerland is economically protected from the consequences of old age, disability, illness, or accident.

Although citizens cannot make direct claims based on this provision, the article nonetheless demonstrates two things. First, it shows the deep-rooted belief in personal responsibility in Switzerland, a belief that extends to health care. Second, it shows that the confederation and the cantons share political responsibility and execute their legislative authority according to their respective competences as stated in the federal constitution.

---

4 Article 41, Federal Constitution of Switzerland.

Regarding policy implementation, there exists a functional division or power sharing between the confederation and the cantons, leaving the cantons the bulk of implementation of federal laws (Linder, 2005, p. 142). This *"federalisme d'exécution"* (Kriesi, 1998, p. 56) has led to a complex governance system where federal authorities depend on cantonal authorities and vice versa.

Among the federal legislative competences enlisted in the constitution referring to health, the articles on health and accident insurance and on the protection of health are the most important. The first[5] gives the confederation the exclusive power to legislate on health insurance. The second[6] refers to public health issues and is a shared responsibility between the confederation and the cantons. From this article on public health, the confederation derives its power to pass bills regulating the pharmaceutical sector and medicines, food, and communicable diseases.

The federal law on health insurance indicates that basic health insurance is mandatory for every person living in Switzerland and specifies that health insurance premiums are to be paid per person (premiums per capita). Consequently, health insurance is not covered by general taxation. Insurers within the mandatory part of the health insurance must be non-profit organizations, although for-profit carriers are permitted for supplementary private health insurance plans. Premiums per capita for the basic health insurance are not paid in relation to health status, income, or other health risk factors but are peer-group based: the same premium per age group (indifferent to gender) and geographical region.

The health insurance law and its regulations are comprehensive, and the basic health insurance benefit package clearly defined. However, political authorities and competences are overlapping and interdependent with the cantons. For example, the cantons decide whether they subsidize health insurance premiums for people in need and to what extent, decisions that then trigger complementary federal subsidies. The cantons also supervise public and university hospitals, which offer medical services that are regulated by federal and cantonal law. Health policy is furthermore intertwined with social, financial, and education policy, each in the sole or concurrent legislative authority of the cantons and the confederation, creating a complex matrix of competencies and jurisdictions.

The confederation is also exclusively responsible for the legislation on vocational training and education comprising all (health) professions not taught at universities. By contrast, the cantons are sovereign in the organization of

---

5 Article 117, Federal Constitution of Switzerland.
6 Article 118, Federal Constitution of Switzerland.

universities and the offering of medical studies. To guarantee a Swiss-wide standard for medical practitioners, however, the confederation supervises the exams of all medical studies at universities as well as the approval of all medical and paramedical professional diplomas gained outside university.

The third governmental layer in the Swiss federation is the municipality. While the political autonomy of municipalities is mentioned in the federal constitution, autonomy and political organization is granted through the cantonal constitution and thus varies from one canton to another. In the typical case, municipalities are responsible for nursing homes and old-age care.

The next section explains in further detail Switzerland's decentralized governance structure by focusing on different aspects of the federal law on health insurance and the relevant actors. This law is a good illustration of where cantonal and centralized federal powers intertwine.

Health Governance and Federalism

Federal Governance Structure and Actors

From the constitutional design there evolved over time a complex institutional framework where political, structure-functional, and legal foundations became highly fragmented yet highly interdependent and where executive federalism structured health governance. Federal authorities have a tendency to create framework legislation not only to spare cantonal legislative sovereignty (Kriesi, 1998, p. 57) but also to reduce deviation in implementation of the federal law (Braun, 2003).

The autonomy in the execution and implementation of federal laws in the context of partial cantonal sovereignty has as a consequence that it is sometimes hard to tell who is responsible and publicly accountable for legislation, regulation, and financing in general, and who is responsible for the execution, implementation, and evaluation of a federal law in particular (Kocher, 2010, p. 138). The governance structure between the federal authorities and the cantons varies from one domain to another and therefore has to be examined case by case (Kriesi, 1998, p. 56).

As a response to complexity, there is a trend at the federal level favouring the centralization of political power in Swiss health affairs (OECD, 2011, p. 140). The OECD and federal authorities have recommended that shared and concurrent responsibilities be reduced through an overarching federal law for health. The aim of such a law would be to set out national objectives and to clarify funding responsibilities and tasks allocated to the three levels of government (Achtermann & Berset, 2006; OCDE, 2006; OECD, 2011). However, the cantons actively resist this trend, as they are very reluctant to give up their powers and responsibilities over health care to the confederation.

Figure 2.1 illustrates the basic governance structure of the Swiss health system. The Federal Office of Public Health (FOPH) plays a key role in health affairs on the national level. In order to better coordinate policy, the FOPH internally created a head office for health policy by the end of 2004. Although the FOPH is the confederation's leading administration branch on health issues, many other federal offices are also involved in health affairs, since health policy is multifunctional and clearly formulated national health objectives are absent. These other offices pursue different goals, with often competing interests (Achtermann & Berset, 2006, p. 59).

FOPH collaborates with these other federal offices in order to coordinate health policies. By working in interdepartmental panels and projects, and using its role as the administrative leader in health affairs, the office tries to bridge the different divisions of the federal administration and their diverging interests. FOPH also works with quasi-independent federal agencies such as Swissmedic.

Swissmedic is the central supervisory authority for therapeutic goods in Switzerland created by a federal law on therapeutics, and it began operating in 2002. Swissmedic, a public not-for-profit corporation owned by the federal government that reports to the Federal Council, has an independent organization, management, and budget. The federal government and service fees fund it. Swissmedic is a good example of the recent trend to centralization: the organization (and the federal law that created it) replaced a long-standing cantonal accord – the Heilmittelkonkordat – between all twenty-six cantons, regulating therapeutic products. This accord was regarded as a jewel of horizontal federalism in health affairs, since only the cantons negotiated the national regulation and the governance structure remained confederal, with the cantons delegating personnel to inspect pharmaceutical production and pass regulations.

During the 1990s, the accord came to be seen as unworkable. As a system of regulation it proved to be too rigid to be adapted to the dynamics of international standardization, in particular of the European Union, and was also not up to date in reference to Swiss-wide needs, such as uniform authorization procedures for pharmaceuticals. However, when the cantons failed to renegotiate a modern accord, they asked the confederation to centralize legislative authority at the national level.

In the health governance structure, the Conference of the Cantonal Ministers of Public Health (CCMPH) plays an important coordinating role between the confederation and the twenty-six cantons. The board consists of seven to ten cantonal health ministers and is elected for a four-year term by the plenum. To prepare the plenary meetings and to deal with actual political issues, the

Figure 2.1 Governance structure of the Swiss health system according to Bundesamt für Gesundheit (2005a, p. 6)

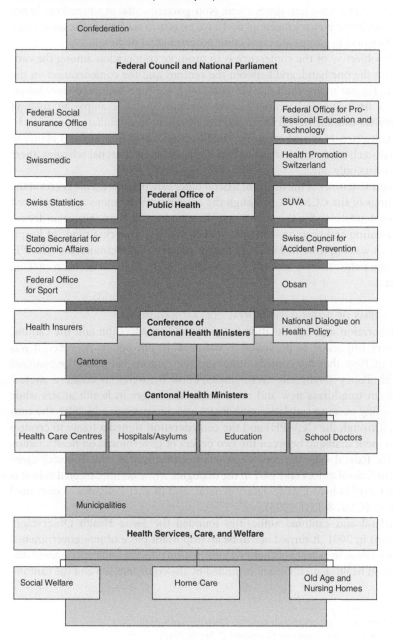

Scheme adapted and translated by the author.

board meets at least four times a year. Non-governmental organizations do not take part in the plenary meetings and have no role in the board. The conference and its working groups are purely intergovernmental bodies.

The objective of the conference is to promote cooperation among the cantons on the one hand, and between the cantons and the confederation on the other. Typical topics the CCMPH deals with are high-tech medicine, hospitals, or financing and tariffs of health services.[7] As an example, in 2008 all twenty-six cantons signed an accord (Interkantonale Vereinbarung zur Hochspezialisierten Medizin) regarding the Swiss-wide organization and planning of high-tech medicine. Instead of twenty-six different cantonal schemes, there now exists only one.

Representatives of the different federal offices are permanent observers at the meetings of the CCMPH. Although the conference's decisions are considered recommendations for the attention of its members, it is an important forum for debating and shaping opinions, such as the new financing mode of hospitals that was implemented in 2012 (explained later). Furthermore, the CCMPH acts as a political actor addressing councillors in the political decision-making process.

NEW FORMS OF INTERGOVERNMENTAL COLLABORATION

Collaboration and coordination between the confederation and the cantons are very important to providing a "national" health policy. However, it was only in 1998 that the confederation and the cantons launched the National Health Policy (Nationale Gesundheitspolitik Schweiz) to create a mutual platform to address new and more costly challenges in health affairs while respecting existing legislative authorities and competences. In 2003, the cantons (through the CCMPH) and the confederation signed a treaty to create a permanent dialogue between the two orders of government on health issues. On the federal side, the confederation's health minister and all health care–related federal offices take part in the dialogue, while on the cantonal side, it is the CCMPH's board, its secretary general, and further delegates of interested cantons (GDK & EDI, 2003).

Federal and cantonal authorities founded the Swiss Health Observatory (Obsan) in 2001. It turned out to be an important piece of intergovernmental collaboration in order to get tailored information relevant for the permanent dialogue on health issues. Obsan[8] is funded by the confederation and the cantons,

---

7 See http://www.gdk-cds.ch/index.php?id=756 (retrieved 6 April 2013).
8 http://www.obsan.admin.ch/en (retrieved 27 August 2017).

is part of the National Health Policy treaty, and is a division of the Swiss Federal Statistical Office (FSO), with a steering committee composed of one member each from the CCMPH, the FOPH, and the FSO. Obsan not only reports to the confederation but also prepares regional or cantonal health reports, according to the requests of the cantons (Achtermann & Berset, 2006, p. 108).

The treaty and the subsequent organization between the confederation and the cantons can be seen as a first step towards nationally coordinated health polices in the fragmented Swiss health system. At the same time, it is a confederal initiative that respects the decentralized nature of the Swiss confederation. However, without changing the decentralized structure of political authorities between the confederation and the cantons in the present, this platform of collaboration could lead to a more centralized health system in the future. The Swiss Health Observatory is thereby a cornerstone, since it prepares available health data in a way that allows for policy coordination across multiple levels of governments.

SHARED COMPETENCES IN PREVENTIVE HEALTH CARE AND HEALTH PROMOTION

An important area of health governance where the cantons and the confederation share legislative power is in preventive health care and health promotion (Bundesamt für Gesundheit, 2007). Because the confederation does not possess an encompassing health law, preventive health care and health promotion is fragmented and decentralized not only vertically but also horizontally within the administration on the federal level.

The confederation's legislative authority regarding preventive health care is restricted to areas such as abatement of communicable diseases, consumption of alcohol and tobacco, protection from chemicals and radiation, preventive health care through environmental protection, and protection of workers. The leading federal administration branch for preventive health care is FOPH, either alone or in collaboration with other federal or cantonal authorities as well as semi-public and private organizations. In order to prevent the spread of HIV, for instance, the FOPH developed successive national awareness campaigns since 1987. Although the FOPH did not have a legal obligation to work together with cantonal authorities, it did seek collaboration with the Swiss AIDS Federation, an umbrella organization uniting cantonal and regional authorities as well as private organizations.[9]

Shared competences between the confederation and the cantons also exist in alcohol addiction prevention. In 2008, the Federal Council launched the four-year national program on alcohol, a program that was extended for

9 http://www.aids.ch/de/ueber-uns/index.php (retrieved 27 August 2017).

another four years in May 2012. The Federal Department of Home Affairs and the Federal Department of Finance were mandated to execute the program. FOPH was subsequently commissioned to develop a coherent policy strategy and implementation to prevent alcohol consumption and addiction. On the federal level, FOPH must work through a fragmented structure, including cooperating with the Swiss Alcohol Board (which collects tax on alcohol as well as inspecting and controlling alcohol production and commerce), a subdivision of the Federal Department of Finance, the Federal Roads Office (alcohol consumption and driving), and the Federal Office of Communications, which bans alcohol advertising (Bundesamt für Gesundheit, 2005b).

An important partner for the supervision and implementation of the program is CCMPH. The twenty-six cantons implement federal law and are responsible (through their legislative authority) for additional prevention strategies in their territories, including regulating advertising, retailers, and alcohol addiction prevention campaigns. Next to their own authority to collect and allocate cantonal taxes, cantons receive 10 per cent from the alcohol levy collected by the confederation on spirits for the purposes of addressing alcohol addiction.

In addition to the confederation and the cantons, there are semi-public, non-profit organizations and private actors active in preventive health care and health promotion (Paccaud & Chiolero, 2010). An interesting case is the foundation Health Promotion Switzerland. The federal law on health insurance states that (private) health insurers have an obligation to promote health. They have to create, together with the cantons, an organization which executes, coordinates, and evaluates measures and programs of health promotion. If the cantons and the health insurers fail in this objective, the confederation has the legal right to step in and take over responsibility for health promotion. Although the confederation has legislative authority deriving from the constitution, in such cases it delegates competencies back to the cantons (and private actors acting under social security law), thereby respecting the principle of subsidiary and decentralized federalism.

Health Promotion Switzerland's board is composed of representatives from Swiss health insurance companies, the cantons, the Swiss Accident Insurance Fund (SUVA),[10] the federal government, medical practitioners and other health care professionals, public health researchers, and

---

10 SUVA is a non-profit company under public law, responsible for preventive health care, work accident insurance, work re-integration, and medical rehabilitation. On the board are representatives of the confederation and employers' and employees' associations.

associations active in health promotion and consumer protection. Selected by the Federal Department of Home Affairs, the board members are appointed for four-year terms. With a full-time staff of thirty employees, Health Promotion Switzerland is financed by a small percentage of health insurance premiums per capita dedicated to health promotion. The Federal Department of Home Affairs sets the annual budget, supervises the foundation, and reports to the responsible committee of the federal parliament about the use of the funds.

Next to the foundation, FOPH runs its own health promotion programs, such as "Food and Motion." Although financed by the budget of the FOPH, these programs are often collaborations between federal agencies (in this case, the Federal Office for Sport and Health Promotion Switzerland) and the cantons (Bundesamt für Gesundheit, 2008). The cantons play a role in staffing, planning, and implementing these strategic public health initiatives.

As these examples of health authority allocation demonstrate, the governance structure for public health activities is decentralized and corporate in its characteristics. Governance in health care and public health occurs through both the federal law on health insurance and national or cantonal public health programs. Collaboration in national health programs often includes not only public authorities but also private for-profit and non-profit organizations. As a consequence the overall governance pattern, cost and financing flows in Swiss health affairs can be confusing and sometimes redundant.

Health Governance Structure at the Cantonal Level

Alongside the Conference of the Cantonal Ministers of Public Health, there exist four regional conferences of cantonal public health ministers: 1) the Suisse Romande and the Tessin (the French- and Italian-speaking parts of Switzerland); 2) Nordwestschweiz (northwestern Switzerland); 3) Ostschweiz and the Principality of Lichtenstein (eastern Switzerland); and 4) Zentralschweiz (central Switzerland).

They possess their own political agenda, financial means, administrative structures, and programs. Within this regional structure of cooperation, the cantons sign numerous regional accords that regulate, for example, hospital planning and the vocational training of non-medical health professions (Achtermann & Berset, 2006, p. 122). The confederation normally is not involved in these political processes and has no authority, unless there exists delegated legislative power to the hands of the confederation or an accord counteracted federal law.

Table 2.1 Intercantonal collaboration in health affairs

Swiss Governmental Tier	Conference of the Cantonal Ministers of Public Health			
	Secretary of the Conference of the Cantonal Ministers of Public Health			
Regional Governmental Tier	Conference of the Cantonal Ministers of Public Health of the Suisse Romande and Tessin (CRASS) Secretary of CRASS	Conference of the Cantonal Ministers of Public Health of Nordwestschweiz	Conference of the Cantonal Ministers of Public Health of Ostschweiz and the Principality of Lichtenstein	Conference of the Cantonal Ministers of Public Health of Zentralschweiz (ZGSDK) Secretary of ZGSDK
Regional Administrative Tier	Standing Group of the Principals of the Cantonal Offices of Public Health		Conference of the Secretaries of the Conference of the Cantonal Ministers of Public Health of Ostschweiz	Health Section Zentralschweiz (Zentralschweizer Fachgruppe Gesundheit)

Source: Drawn from Achtermann and Berset (2006, p. 78), translated by the author

Financing Sources of the Swiss Health System – the Macro Financial Streams

The total cost of the health system as a percentage of the gross domestic product (GDP) was 10.9 per cent in 2012.[11] Hospitals accounted for about 37.5 per cent of total health spending, outpatient providers (e.g., private medical practitioners) for 30.3 per cent, nursing homes for 13.3 per cent, institutions for disabled persons for 4.1 per cent,[12] retail sale of pharmaceuticals and therapeutic instruments for 8.2 per cent, and the administrative costs and expenditures on health and accident prevention borne by the insurers (4 per cent), by the state (1.6 per cent), and by private non-profit health leagues (1.1 per cent). Regarding financing sources in the health system, the confederation paid 3.8 billion Swiss francs (the bulk of it for health insurance premium subsidies) while the cantons paid 15.2 billion and the municipalities 3.0 billion in 2012. Private households

---

11 Swiss Statistics, https://www.bfs.admin.ch/bfs/portal/en/index/themen/14/05/blank/key/ueberblick.html (retrieved 9 January 2014).

12 Ibid.

allocated 41.6 billion Swiss francs to the financing of the health system, and corporations an additional 4.3 billion francs through social and private health insurances regimes.[13]

Although the law on health insurance[14] is complex and premiums are expensive, Swiss citizens support the overall approach.[15] This may be due to the high quality of the Swiss health system (OECD, 2011), but it is also because the strong emphasis on individual health responsibility is counterbalanced by premium subsidies for the poor paid by the state (Longchamp, Kocher, Tschöpe, Deller, & Portmann, 2012, p. 6). Individual responsibility therefore goes along with solidarity to build broad public support for the design and financing of the health system.

HEALTH INSURANCE PREMIUMS AND CANTONAL RELIEF PROGRAMS

In 2010, about 2.3 million Swiss citizens, 29.8 per cent of all insured people in the country, received means-tested subsidies to pay their health insurance premiums, worth 4 billion Swiss francs (Kägi, Frey, Säuberli, Feer, & Koch, 2012, p. X). Since the 1980s, health insurance premiums per capita have been a major bone of contention between Social Democrats (SP) on the one hand and parts of the Christian-Democratic Party (CVP) as well as the Radical Party (FDP) and People's Party (SVP) on the other (Braun & Uhlmann, 2009; Uhlmann & Braun, 2011). To find a political compromise on health system reform that would satisfy the SP, it was important to subsidize the health insurance holder (in particular families, low-income households, and the elderly). At the same time it was necessary to keep the policy instrument of individual premiums per capita to satisfy the other parties. The result was means-tested health premium subsidies.

The subsidization of health premiums was left to the authority of the cantons. The confederation financially assists the cantons with an annual contribution of 7.5 per cent of the gross expenses incurred by the mandatory health insurance. Because of a change in co-financing due to a new formula for federal equalization introduced in 2008, the cantons increased their rate of subsidization from 34 per cent to 49 per cent (Kägi et al., 2012, p. X).

The cantonal subsidy schemes differ considerably (Balthasar, 2003; Balthasar, 2005) because of varying determinations of premium reductions, the criteria for eligibility, deadlines for applications, and the modes of relief payments by cantons (Balthasar, Bieri, & Müller, 2005, p. 31). However, since the federal

---

13 Ibid.
14 Federal law on health insurance (Bundesgesetz über die Krankenversicherung, SR 832.10), from 18 March 1994 (1 January 2012).
15 Consumer survey on the federal law on health insurance: http://www.presseportal.ch/ pm/100003671/100707527 (retrieved 10 April 2013).

law on health insurance in 1996, the modes of cantonal relief programs have become more aligned. Whereas in the past there were a great variety of schemes, now the cantonal subsidy programs can be classified into three basic models: 1) a single percentage model (ten cantons); 2) a stage model[16] (eight cantons); and 3) a hybrid model using both percentages and stages (eight cantons) (Kägi et al., 2012, p. XI).

The Federal Council set a guideline that the premium charge for each household's income should not exceed 6 to 8 per cent Swiss-wide (Kägi et al., 2012, p. XIII). However, with the different cantonal premium relief programs in place, this objective could not be attained in 2010, although a total of 4.04 billion Swiss francs were allocated to subsidy health insurance premiums – 2,072 million by the cantons and 1,975 million by the confederation (Kägi et al., 2012). The average financial burden for a household varied according to the size and makeup of the respective households, from 7 to 13 per cent (Kägi et al., 2012, p. XIII). This means that equity in the financing of the health insurance system has not been attained so far.

Decision Space

According to Bossert (1998, p. 1514), decision space is the range of choice available to local decision makers along functional dimensions such as financing, service organization, human resources, targeting, and governance. What we have seen in the Swiss health system so far is that the decision space in health affairs for the cantons varies substantially by function.

Finance

In terms of health care system financing, almost two-thirds of financing comes from private households. This includes premiums per capita for the mandatory health insurance, private health insurance premiums, and out-of-pocket payments. Figure 2.2 demonstrates that the cantons are, by far, the most important state actors in terms of control over the allocation of fiscal resources. In contrast to the 21 per cent of cantonal financing, the 6 per cent and 4 per cent

---

16 In the stage model different classes of income are defined to evaluate the eligible persons. According to the different classes, a fixed amount is paid to subsidize the health insurance premium. In contrast to the percentage model, which aims for a guiding premium in reference to the income, e.g., 8 per cent, and consequently varies in individual subsidies, stage-model-related subsidies are fixed according to the respective income class (see Kägi et al., 2012, p. XI).

Figure 2.2 Financing sources of the Swiss health system, 2010, in percentage of total costs (62.5 billion Swiss francs)

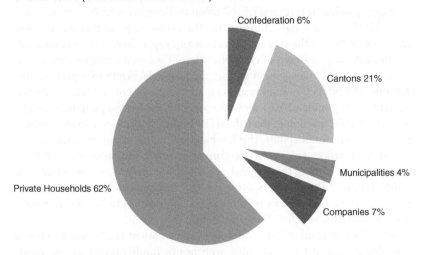

Confederation 6%

Cantons 21%

Municipalities 4%

Companies 7%

Private Households 62%

Author's graph according to Bundesamt für Statistik (2012).

of the confederation and the municipalities, respectively, show their lesser importance.

Cantons are free to choose where and how to allocate their health budgets. Since the confederation has only limited administrative resources, the cantons most often implement and execute federal legislation. However, in comparison to the total cantonal health spending, costs and financial transfers play only a minor role (see Kanton Basel-Stadt, 2011, p. 52, for an example). A rare ear-marked health transfer to the cantons is the 10 per cent share of the federal alcohol levy. According to the federal constitution, the share is meant to coun-teract alcohol (drug) addiction and conduct preventive health care. Although the transfer is earmarked, the cantons are quite free in its usage and act as they think best to fulfil this obligation. In conclusion, the cantonal decision space on financing is wide.

Service Organization

Although the coverage of health care services is regulated by the federal law on health insurance, the planning and coordination of health care provisioning (inpa-tient, ambulant, and emergency services in hospitals) is a classic prerogative of the cantons (Bundesrat, 2004, p. 5555) and explicitly mentioned in the federal law itself.[17] This includes the full spectrum of private and public hospitals providing acute care, psychiatric care, and rehabilitation and long-term health care services.

Until 2009 the cantonal authorities ran the public hospitals themselves. They were responsible for the strategic direction and supervision of public hospitals as well as the appointment of chief physicians. Cantonal laws also defined the operative hospital management and set the hospitals' health care provisioning planning, the budget, human resources, and employment conditions (Berger, Bienlein, & Wegmüller, 2010). However, in 2009, the federal parliament implemented a partial revision of the federal law on health insurance to alter financing mechanisms for hospitals. This law has had four main policy consequences.

First, the revision triggered a transformation process in financing itself: from financing and planning the hospital as a whole to reimbursing and purchasing health services.[18] The change occurred via the introduction of diagnosis-related groups (DRGs). Lump sums paid for Swiss DRG cases are based on uniform Swiss-wide tariffs, which did not exist before the reform.

Second, since January 2012, cantons where a patient resides have to pay at least 55 per cent of DRG flat rates, with health funds making up the difference. While federal law regulates this cantonal minimum percentage, cantons are free to contribute above the 55 per cent threshold. This means that cantons no longer pay for all the investments in hospital infrastructure and personnel but instead cost-share with health insurers via DRGs. Since the cantons are no longer responsible for either the appointment of chief medical personnel or direct investments in infrastructure, in their new role, the cantons supervise and monitor rather than manage hospitals.

Third, with the revision, the federal law specified pre-existing hospital licensing and planning criteria for the cantons. The cantons still do the cantonal provisioning planning. However, they have to take into account the licensing and planning criteria (for adequate medical care, appropriate qualified personnel, suitable medical infrastructure, and pharmaceutical provisioning, quality, and cost-effectiveness) that are set by the federal law and the Federal Council. To some extent, the Federal Council supervises the cantonal planning and asks for corrections if the cantonal planning is deemed inadequate. This is the case, for example, when the federal government determines that there is too much inpatient capacity, or criticizes the absence of clear service-level agreements between

---

17 Article 39, federal law on health insurance (Bundesgesetz über die Krankenversicherung, SR 832.10), from 18 March 1994 (1 January 2012).

18 FOPH, https://archive.is/1cN3Q (retrieved 18 April 2013).

hospitals and the cantonal government.[19] Even though there is supervision from the Federal Council, the CCMPH plays an important role for the cantonal and intercantonal planning of inpatient services. CCMPH has published recommendations for hospital planning for the cantons (GDK, 2009) and coordinates planning among cantons (GDK, 2013). On the national level, CCMPH has consistently influenced health insurance reform and service organization legislation in favour of the cantons' interests (GDK, 2006; GDK, 2007).

Fourth, with the revision of the federal law on health insurance, competition became a stronger structuring element in the organization of hospital services. Patients, benefitting from the basic health insurance package, were empowered to choose among hospitals throughout Switzerland as long as the hospitals are on a planning list set up by the cantons. Cantonal governments and health insurance companies are now obligated by the federal law to reimburse costs generated by these hospital stays. With this empowerment of "consumers," the market was strengthened at the expense, to some extent, of cantonal planning authority.

As a reaction to this change of federal legislation, most of the cantonal authorities granted more autonomy and entrepreneurial freedom to public hospitals to organize health services according to consumers' choice. However, the legal status and accompanying entrepreneurial freedom of public hospitals varies among cantons since the cantons control the legal status of hospitals.

Although cantonal decision space has grown smaller, the cantons nonetheless supervise and control hospitals, including the organization of inpatient health services, in their respective territories by contractual agreements. As their power in hospital affairs remains strong (Berger et al., 2010, p. 376), cantonal decision space still can be labelled wide. In contrast, outpatient services are regulated at the national level. Since the federal law on health insurance standardizes the uniform benefit package of mandated health insurance, the canton's range of choice in defining the benefit package is narrow.

Cantons are responsible for the occupational licensing and the practice of medical and paramedical professions (Bundesamt für Gesundheit, 2005a). Medical practitioners, dentists, and physical therapists need to get allowances from cantonal authorities – not the confederation – to practice their profession on the territory of the respective canton. The same applies to labour and contract agreements and the organization of health services. To be able to bill

19 See as an example the case of the canton Tessin: https://www.ejpd.admin.ch/content/ejpd/de/home/dokumentation/mi/2000/2000-05-031.html (retrieved 19 April 2013).

health services covered by the federal law on health insurance, health care providers have to negotiate contracts on tariffs and prices with health funds. These tariffs are negotiated for the mandatory benefit package where health funds operate on a not-for-profit basis. Normally the professions' and health insurers' umbrella organizations succeed in agreeing upon tariffs and prices. Cantonal authorities, or the confederation for nationwide agreements, would step in to set tariffs only if these partners failed. Nonetheless, cantons and the confederation have the authority to dictate tariffs and prices in order to guarantee the provisioning of health services. In regard to the federal law on health insurance, there exist over 100 labour agreements, which define tariffs, prices, and payment modes for different health professions and providers (Wyler, 2010, p. 414). All of these contracts have to be approved by cantonal – or, for national tariffs, federal – authorities. Here, there is no obvious trend towards greater centralization.

Access Rules and Human Resources

The federal government sets the basic access rules including the mandatory requirement for health insurance as well as the benefit package for the compulsory insurance. Cantons and health insurance companies cannot change access rules and are required to follow federal regulations. However, cantons can use their legislative authority in social policies related to health (health premium relief programs, family assistance schemes, mammography screening, etc.) for targeting groups they want to support. Consequently, decision space is narrow for mandatory health insurance but wide for related social programs.

Cantons have a wide decision space concerning human resources. Although the federal Swiss Code of Obligations regulates employer-employee relationships under private law, Article 342 of the law grants wide autonomy to federal and cantonal authorities to establish special labour conditions. As a result, there are twenty-seven different human resources acts in Switzerland.[20] Cantonal authorities can decide upon salary ranges, contracting non-permanent staff, and employment conditions, including hiring and firing.[21] Limitations in the decision space occur in social insurance for old age, unemployment, and

---

20 See for an overview of the federal and cantonal corpus juris in reference to the Human Resources Acts, https://www.oeffentliches-personalrecht.ch/gesetzliche-grundlage (retrieved 12 April 13).

21 See as an example Human Resources Act Canton Basel-Town (Personalgesetz Kanton Basel-Stadt vom 17. November 1999, Stand 1. January 2012): http://www.gesetzessammlung.bs.ch/frontend/versions/1918 (retrieved 12 April 13).

disability, since a certain percentage of the wages are used to finance these social insurance plans, which are regulated by federal law. Superannuation plans of permanent staff, too, can be set up by each canton individually. However, cantonal authorities have to follow federal regulation in order to financially protect these plans. Although there are limitations, the cantonal decision space in human resources remains wide.

Governance Rules

As demonstrated in Figures 2.1 and 2.2, governance in Swiss health affairs is based on a multitude of actors at three levels of governments, and no encompassing framework on health legislation exists at the national level. Nevertheless, the cantons' overall health governance decision space is shrinking and now oscillates between wide and moderate. In some cases it remains wide, particularly when intercantonal accords, intergovernmental bodies, or facility boards are involved, since these governance structures are set up by the cantons. In this sense, it also remains wide regarding cantonal health offices and the governance rules of community and citizens' participation in cantonal health affairs. However, some cantonal decision space is narrow. When federal law replaced cantonal accord prerogative in the 1990s, the cantons' previously wide pharmaceutical governance structure narrowed. For example, federal law regulates the board of Swissmedic, and cantonal authorities now only propose a maximum of three (out of seven) board members to the Federal Council. In addition to appointing Swissmedic's president and director, the Council also has discretion to reject any of the cantonal candidates for the board.

In other governance areas, such as hospital planning, cantons still have a wide decision space, and they intend to keep this sphere of influence. In reforming the federal law on health insurance, the Conference of Cantonal Public Health Ministers played an active role to shape policy change in their favour. And, although there exists federal legislation regarding hospitals, cantonal authorities nonetheless enjoy substantial decision space in the setup of the governance structure for inpatient and acute care, highly specialized medical treatment, and the negotiation and supervision of service-level agreements with hospitals. Furthermore, as was demonstrated, cantonal authorities enjoy the freedom to negotiate and sign intercantonal accords on hospital planning and vocational training. Cantons also use regional conferences of cantonal public health ministers and their legislative competences to conclude intergovernmental health agreements (Achtermann & Berset, 2006, pp. 122–8). Both intercantonal accords and intergovernmental health agreements are cornerstones of the cantonal health governance architecture.

Figure 2.3 Cantonal decision space according to functional dimension

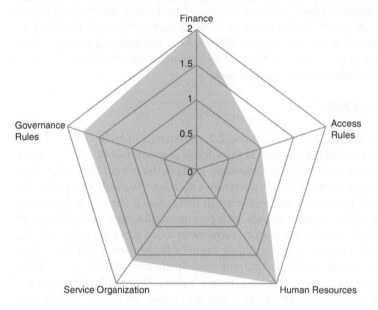

Figure 2.3 demonstrates the cantonal decision space according to various functional dimensions. Cantonal decision space in finance, access rules, human resources, service organization, and governance rules is substantial. This means decentralization is high and cantons still have an important say in health affairs.

Most federal restrictions occur in the dimension of access rules. This is not surprising given that the equity dimension of the health system was one of the most important (and controversial) issues in the 1994 reform of the federal law on health insurance – and a cornerstone of Social Democratic health policy. Social Democrats sought to alter the pre-existing federal law on health insurance in favour of more solidarity, social justice, and equity. The party pursued these goals by popular initiatives, proposing reforms in Parliament and in the Federal Council (Uhlmann & Braun, 2011). With the reform, access rules to the health insurance were standardized nationally, including access to a uniform basic benefit package, in order to guarantee health equity.

In contrast, the cantons' financial decision space is wide. Since the cantons have the primarily power to levy taxes, they also have considerable discretion over the allocation of health spending. The same is true for human resources. As was demonstrated, cantons enjoy wide decision space over cantonal personnel in terms of legislation, recruitment, remuneration, and task allocation.

The cantons' governance decision space can be gauged as wide, too. Overall, cantonal decision space in the Swiss health system is substantial.

Conclusion and Trend Delineation

Decentralization of power and quasi-sovereignty of the cantons remains the principal structuring feature of Swiss federalism. In the beginning (1848), the legislative power of the confederation in health affairs was very limited and led to the emergence of twenty-six cantonal health systems along with a few select federal health competences. Now, the confederation is involved in the health system in many ways. Nevertheless, the cantons are the holders of residual legislative powers and have an important role in financing, organizing, and delivering health care (OCDE, 2006; OECD, 2011). This means the health system is still highly decentralized to the cantonal level, with only a little power left to the municipalities.

Coordination and cooperation in this system occurs through regional and national intergovernmental bodies, which permit cantonal authorities to work together in a consensus-based partnership. Apart from the horizontal cooperation, CCMPH is the main member states' advocacy body in collaboration with the confederation. However, coordination in health affairs between the confederation and the cantons is more the exception than the rule.

The trend in governance of the health system is towards some increased centralization, as the canton decision space in a few areas of health care has shrunk modestly. As was argued, equity considerations led to harmonization at the national level in the case of the federal law on health insurance in 1994. In 2002, financial concerns and pressure of international standardization caused centralization in the case of the cantonal accord about therapeutic products and pharmaceuticals, while vocational training and education (including for health professionals) was concentrated in the legislative authority of the confederation. There also now exists federal supervision in the case of cantonal hospital planning. Furthermore, the introduction of market mechanisms in the organization and management of hospitals and the provisioning of inpatient care in 2012 led to a modest weakening of the cantonal governing power in health affairs.

In most cases, cantons are very reluctant to hand over their legislative power in health affairs to the confederation. While Switzerland remains highly decentralized in terms of its health system, cantonal authorities will only succeed in keeping their decision space if they can prove to their electorate that they are able to provide cost-efficient health services of good quality, taking into account a certain degree of solidarity. Otherwise, the cantons may eventually see a continued and perhaps far more radical shift of their legislative power to the central government.

Appendix

Table 2.2 Cantonal decision space according to finance, service organization, human resources, access rules, and governance rules (Bossert, 1998)

Function	Indicator	Range of Choice		
		Narrow	Moderate	Wide
Financing				
Sources of revenue	% of total (state) health spending			Strong health financing power in contrast to confederation and municipalities
Expenditure allocation	% of cantonal spending explicitly earmarked by federal government			Earmarking very marginal and very limited oversight
Service organization and delivery				
Hospital autonomy	Range of autonomy for hospitals			No limits
Hospital planning and provisioning	Range of authority in hospital planning			Few limits: wide constitutional planning authority reduced according to guideline criteria set by federal law and the Federal Council
Insurance plans	Specificity of norms for cantonal programs	Mandatory health insurance plans are standardized by federal law and uniform Swiss-wide		
Required programs (Alcohol)	Specificity of norms for cantonal programs			No limits on diversity of cantonal alcohol addiction prevention programs; no specified norms

Human resources		
Salaries	Choice of salary range	No limits
Contracting	Contracting non-permanent staff	No limits
Civil service	Hiring and firing	No limits
Labour agreements	Range of authority in approval of labour agreements	All cantonal labour agreements have to approved by cantonal authorities
Access rules		
Health insurance	Extent to which subpopulations or services can be targeted	Uniform benefit package to all residents
Health-related social policy	Extent to which subpopulations or services can be targeted	Cantons enjoy wide freedom to define targeting groups
Governance rules		
Federal health facility boards	Size and composition of boards	Size and boards' composition vary according to federal law, and agreements between the confederation and the cantons (Swissmedic, Obsan, etc.)
Intercantonal accords (concordat) and subsequent intercantonal health facility boards	Size and composition of boards	Very few limits: treaties are not allowed to contradict federal law
Cantonal health offices	Size and composition of cantonal health offices	No limits
Community participation	Size, number, composition, and role of participation	No limits

REFERENCES

Achtermann, W., & Berset, C. (2006). *Gesundheitspolitiken in der Schweiz – Potential für eine nationale Gesundheitspolitik: Analyse und Perspektiven.* Bern, Switzerland: Bundesamt für Gesundheit.

Balthasar, A. (2003). Prämienverbilligung im Krankenversicherungsgesetz: Vollzugsföderalismus und sekundäre Harmonisierung. *Sonderheft Föderalismus der Schweizerische Zeitschrift für Politikwissenschaft, herausgegeben von Adrian Vatter und Sonja Wälti, 2003*(1), 335–54.

Balthasar, A. (2005). *Die Prämienverbilligung in den Kantonen: Übersicht über Bemessungsgrundlagen, Berechnungsmodelle und Bagatellgrenzen in den 16 Kantonen.* Lucerne, Switzerland: Interface.

Balthasar, A., Bieri, O., & Müller, F. (2005). *Monitoring 2004: Die sozialpolitische Wirksamkeit der Prämienverbilligung in den Kantonen.* Bern, Switzerland: Bundesamt für Gesundheit/Interface Institut für Politikstudien.

Berger, S., Bienlein, M., & Wegmüller, B. (2010). Spitäler. In G. Kocher & W. Oggier (Eds.), *Gesundheitswesen Schweiz 2010–2012: Eine aktuelle Übersicht* (pp. 373–89). Bern, Switzerland: Verlag Hans Huber.

Bossert, T. (1998). Analyzing the decentralization of health systems in developing countries: Decision space, innovation and performance. *Social Science & Medicine, 47*(10), 1513–27.

Braun, D. (2003). Dezentraler und unitarischer Föderalismus: Die Schweiz und Deutschland im Vergleich. *Schweizerische Zeitschrift für Politikwissenschaft, 9*(1), 57–89.

Braun, D., & Uhlmann, B. (2009). Explaining policy stability and change in Swiss health care reform. *Schweizerische Zeitschrift für Politikwissenschaft, 15*(2), 205–40.

Bundesamt für Gesundheit. (2005a). *Das schweizerische Gesundheitswesen.* Bern, Switzerland: Bundesamt für Gesundheit.

Bundesamt für Gesundheit. (2005b). *Prävention und Gesundheitsförderung in der Schweiz – Stand: Oktober 2005: B. f. Gesundheit.* Bern, Switzerland: Bundesamt für Gesundheit.

Bundesamt für Gesundheit. (2007). *Prävention und Gesundheitsförderung in der Schweiz.* Bern, Switzerland: Bundesamt für Gesundheit.

Bundesamt für Gesundheit. (2008). *Nationales Programm Ernährung und Bewegung 2008–2012 (NPEB 2008–2012).* Bern, Switzerland: Bundesamt für Gesundheit.

Bundesamt für Statistik. (2012). *Kosten und Finanzierung des Gesundheitswesens 2010 (provisorisch): EDI.* Bern, Switzerland: Bundesamt für Statistik.

Bundesrat. (2004, September). Botschaft betreffend die Änderung des Bundesgesetzes über die Krankenversicherung (Spitalfinanzierung) vom 15. Bern, Switzerland, Schweizerische Bundeskanzlei.

GDK. (2006). Rapport annuel – Jahresbericht 2006. Bern, Switzerland, Schweizerische Konferenz der kantonalen Gesundheitsdirektorinnen und -direktoren.

GDK. (2007). Rapport annuel – Jahresbericht 2007. Bern, Switzerland, Schweizerische Konferenz der kantonalen Gesundheitsdirektorinnen und -direktoren.

GDK. (2009). Empfehlungen der GDK zur Spitalplanung unter Berücksichtigung der KVG-Revision zur Spitalfinanzierung vom 21.12.2007. Bern, Switzerland, Schweizerische Konferenz der kantonalen Gesundheitsdirektorinnen und -direktoren.

GDK. (2013). Übersicht kantonale Spitallisten und Spitaltarife 2012/2013. Bern, Switzerland, Schweizerische Konferenz der kantonalen Gesundheitsdirektorinnen und -direktoren.

GDK & EDI. (2003). Vereinbarung zwischen der Schweizerischen Konferenz der kantonalen Gesundheitsdirektorinnen und -direktoren (GDK) und der Schweizerischen Eidgenossenschaft (Bund) vertreten durch das Eidg. Departement des Innern (EDI). Bern, Switzerland, Die Schweizerische Eidgenossenschaft.

Hueglin, T.O., & Fenna, A. (2005). *Comparative federalism: A systematic inquiry.* Toronto, ON: University of Toronto Press.

Immergut, E.M. (1990). Institutions, veto points, and policy results: A comparative analysis of health care. *Journal of Public Policy, 10*(4), 391–416.

Immergut, E.M. (1992). *Health politics: Interests and institutions in Western Europe.* Cambridge, UK: Cambridge University Press.

Kägi, W., Frey, M., Säuberli, C., Feer, M., & Koch, P. (2012). Monitoring 2010. Wirksamkeit der Prämienverbilligung. Bern, Basel, Bundesamt für Gesundheit/ B,S,S. Volkswirtschaftliche Beratung AG Basel.

Kanton Basel-Stadt. (2011). *Bericht zum Budget 2012: Regierungsrat.* Basel, Switzerland: Kanton Basel-Stadt.

Kocher, G. (2010). *Kompetenz- und Aufgabenteilung Bund – Kantone – Gemeinden.* In G. Kocher and W. Oggier (Eds.), *Gesundheitswesen Schweiz 2010–2012: Eine aktuelle Übersicht* (pp. 133–44). Bern, Switzerland: Verlag Hans Huber.

Kriesi, H. (1998). *Le système politique suisse.* Paris, FR: Economica.

Kriesi, H. (1999). *Introduction: State formation and nation building in the Swiss case.* In H. Kriesi, K. Armingeon, H. Siegrist, & A. Wimmer (Eds.), *Nation and national identity: The European experience in perspective* (pp. 13–28). Chur, Switzerland: Verlag Rüegger.

Lijphart, A. (1999). *Patterns of democracy: Government forms and performance in thirty-six countries.* New Haven, CT: Yale University Press.

Linder, W. (2005). *Schweizerische Demokratie: Institutionen, Prozesse, Perspektiven (2. Auflage).* Bern, Switzerland: Haupt.

Linder, W., & Steffen, I. (2007). Political culture. In U. Klöti, P. Knoepfel, H. Kriesi, W. Linder, & Y. Papadopoulos (Eds.), *Handbook of Swiss politics* (2nd ed.) (pp. 15–34). Zürich, Switzerland: NZZ Verlag.

Longchamp, C., Kocher, J.P., Tschöpe, S., Deller, S., & Portmann, A. (2012). Gesundheitspolitik im veränderten Umfeld. Schlussbericht zum Gesundheitsmonitor 2012. Bern, gfs.bern.

OCDE. (2006). Examens de l'OCDE des systèmes de santé - Suisse. Paris, FR: OECD.

OECD. (2011). OECD reviews of health systems: Switzerland. Paris, FR: OECD.

Paccaud, F., & Chiolero, A. (2010). Prävention, Gesundheitsförderung und Public Health. In G. Kocher and W. Oggier (Eds.), Gesundheitswesen Schweiz 2010–2012: Eine aktuelle Übersicht (pp. 309–19). Bern, Switzerland: Verlag Hans Huber.

Papadopoulos, Y. (1995). Analysis of functions and dysfunctions of direct democracy: Top-down and bottom-up perspectives. Politics & Society, 23(4), 421–48.

Requejo, F. (2006). Federalism and democracy: The case of minority nations: A federalist deficit. Barcelona, Spain: University of Pompeu Fabra.

Sciarini, P. (2007). The decision-making process. In U. Klöti, P. Knoepfel, H. Kriesi, W. Linder, & Y. Papadopoulos (Eds.), Handbook of Swiss politics (2nd ed.) (pp. 465–500). Zürich, Switzerland: NZZ Verlag.

Tsebelis, G. (2002). Federalism and veto players. In U. Wagschal and H. Rentsch (Eds.), Der Preis des Föderalismus (pp. 295–318). Zürich, Switzerland: Orell Füssli.

Uhlmann, B., & Braun, D. (2011). Die Schweizerische Krankenversicherungspolitik zwischen Veränderung und Stillstand. Zürich, Switzerland: Rüegger Verlag.

Wyler, D. (2010). Tarife. In G. Kocher and W. Oggier (Eds.), Gesundheitswesen Schweiz 2010–2012: Eine aktuelle Übersicht, 413–21. Bern, Switzerland: Verlag Hans Huber.

Chapter Three

Health Care in Canada: Interdependence and Independence

GREGORY P. MARCHILDON

Structural Features of the Canadian Federation

Canada is both a federation and a multinational polity with a minority nation (Québécois) that forms the majority population in one province (Québec). This, more than any other single fact, has produced one of the most decentralized federations in the world. And similar to other multinational federations or quasi-federations such as India and Spain, there is some constitutional asymmetry in the powers and responsibilities exercised by provincial governments. With a provincial party system that is distinct from that at the national level, as well as two secessionist parties – one in Québec and one at the federal level that runs candidates solely in Québec – decentralization is built into the political DNA of the country (Marchildon, 2009). Therefore, the relative decentralization of publicly financed health care must be put into the context of a federal polity that is already highly decentralized (Marchildon, 2013a).

Requejo (2010) uses a 20-point scale to assess the level of decentralization according to legislative authority in key policy areas, executive-administrative powers, foreign policy, and fiscal autonomy to compare nineteen federations in the world. Based on this scale, Canada was tied with Bosnia-Herzegovina as the most decentralized federations in this group. Of even greater interest is the fact that the Canadian provinces are scored, by a considerable margin, as the most fiscally autonomous subnational states in the world, a result consistent with earlier evaluations of fiscal decentralization (Marchildon, 1995; Requejo, 2010).

Introduction to Canadian Federation and Health System Decentralization

A constitutional monarchy based on a British-style parliamentary system, Canada has only two constitutionally recognized orders of government. The first order is the central or "federal" government, while the second and constitutionally equal order of government consists of the ten provincial governments that bear the principal policy and administrative responsibility for a range of social policy programs and services, including the majority of publicly financed health services. Local and municipal governments are treated as "creatures" of the provinces, with delegated lawmaking, limited revenue-raising capacities, and restricted responsibilities for health (e.g., health and safety regulation of food services) and almost no responsibility for health care.

Medically necessary hospital and medical services are free at the point of service for all provincial residents through single-payer coverage plans individually administered by provincial governments. Through conditional transfers to the provinces, the federal government encourages the maintenance of key national dimensions such as portability and universality by the provincial government, which is responsible for administering and delivering these services, creating the semblance of a national health system.

Beyond the universal basket of hospital and medical (i.e., physician) services, provincial governments subsidize or provide other health goods and services, including what are known as extended health benefits such as some prescription drug coverage and subsidies for long-term care services (facility-based nursing care) and home care. These provincial programs generally target subpopulations on the basis of age or income. The federal government also subsidizes or provides services to targeted subpopulations including registered Indians (First Nations) and Inuit residents, members of the Armed Forces, veterans, inmates in federal penitentiaries, and eligible refugee claimants. In addition, the federal government has important responsibilities in the domains of public health, pharmaceutical regulation, health-related research, and health data collection.

However, given the policy interdependencies and overlaps in health care, both the federal and provincial governments have developed numerous collaborative processes, such as councils and working groups, established by federal and provincial ministers and deputy ministers of health. In addition, possibly to an extent that surpasses similar efforts in other federations, provincial and federal governments, acting together, have established a number of specialized intergovernmental agencies and organizations to manage these policy interdependencies and overlaps.

This chapter analyses the extent of health system decentralization as well as current trends, beginning with an examination of the structural features of the Canadian federation. Health system decentralization is then examined in terms of decision space choice and capacity in various domains: governance, financing (including federal transfers to the provinces), and human resource planning. This section concludes with a description of the intergovernmental

Figure 3.1 Map of Canada

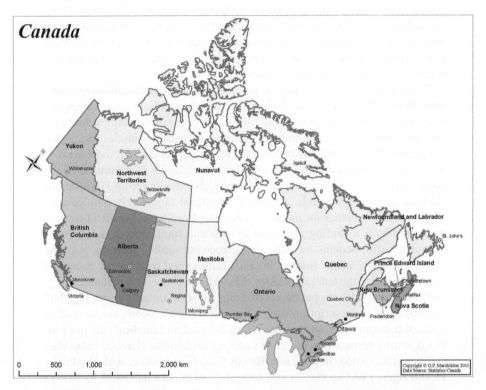

culture, processes, and organizations that typify the relationship between the provincial and federal governments as the stewards of the Canadian health system. The final section examines the trends in health system decentralization and centralization in Canada. Although these trends are presented within their historical context, the focus is on major changes since 2000.

Constitutional Authority and Health System Organization

The constitution, with its division of powers and responsibilities among governments, is the essential starting point in any discussion of the structural dimensions of any federation. In the Canadian case, this division of powers and responsibilities was formulated in the 1860s and, with only a modest amendment in 1982, has remained the same for the past century and a half. As a consequence, health and health care were not addressed as distinct subjects in the

original constitution, and the only explicit mention involved provincial jurisdiction over hospital and psychiatric institutions (Fierlbeck & Palley, 2015).
Beyond this, authority can only be inferred from a number of general provisions in the constitution, but subsequent judicial decisions support the view
that the provinces have primary, but not exclusive, jurisdiction over health and
health care (Braën, 2004; Leeson, 2004).

This is partly because the federal government has jurisdiction over specific
areas that, while not directly connected to health care, have taken on greater
relevance to this domain over time. One example is federal responsibility for
"Indians," which has come to mean Indians as registered under the Indian
Act, many of whom still live on reserves located in rural and remote areas of
the country, as well as Inuit, the majority of whom live in communities on the
coast of the Arctic Ocean and who are considered distinct from First Nations
(Indian) groups as a whole. Although provincial (and territorial) governments provide coverage for medically necessary hospital and medical services
for all residents including registered Indians and Inuit, they do not provide
extended health benefits for individuals receiving similar coverage from the
Government of Canada. Instead, the First Nations and Inuit Health Branch of
Health Canada – the federal ministry of health – provides those eligible Indigenous residents with supplemental coverage for "non-insured health benefits"
(NIHB) such as prescription drugs, dental care, and vision care, as well as
medical transportation so they can access hospital and medical care not provided in their respective reserves or northern settlements (Lavoie, 2004; Marchildon et al., 2015). In addition, Health Canada in concert with the Public
Health Agency of Canada – a new federal department established in 2003 to
address pan-Canadian issues of population health, public health surveillance,
and monitoring – also fund a number of population health and community
health programs in First Nations and Inuit communities.

In addition, the federal government has jurisdiction over patents, including
pharmaceutical patents, and therefore the constitutional ability to regulate patented drug prices, which it does through the Patented Medicine Prices Review
Board (PMPRB). The federal government is also responsible for regulating the
safety and efficacy of therapeutic products such as medical devices, pharmaceuticals, and natural health products. Finally, the federal government plays a
critical role in health research through its funding of the Canadian Institutes
of Health Research (CIHR), 70 per cent of which is allocated to investigator-
driven research and 30 per cent to strategic objectives set by CIHR's governing council. This research activity is supported by an extensive infrastructure
for health data provided by Statistics Canada and its periodic health surveys.
The federal government also contributes the lion's share of funding to the

Canadian Institute for Health Information (CIHI), the principal depository for provincial and territorial administrative health data. While these federal activities constitute only 3.5 per cent of total health spending in Canada, they involve critical stewardship responsibilities at the very apex of the health system (Marchildon, 2012).

Figure 3.2 is a constitutional-political organization chart of the Canadian health system. Highly simplified, this chart focuses on the roles, responsibilities, and accountabilities of the federal and provincial governments. Even though the three territorial governments in northern Canada do not exercise the constitutional autonomy of the provinces, they are included in Figure 3.2 because they behave like provinces in terms of their policy and program responsibilities in health care. However, given this constitutional difference, the discussion that follows will be limited to the two constitutionally recognized orders of governments – provincial and federal (Marchildon, 2013a).

As shown in Figure 3.2, most of the day-to-day responsibility of administering publicly funded health services is in the hands of the provinces. In particular, they are responsible for administering single-payer coverage for medically necessary hospital and medical services that must meet the five criteria – public administration, comprehensiveness, universality, portability, and accessibility – as defined under the federal Canada Health Act. These criteria or national dimensions are "enforced" through the threat of withdrawal of federal transfer money from the provinces. Since 1978, the cash value of this federal transfer has fluctuated between 25 and 30 per cent of total provincial expenditures on hospital and physician expenditures (Romanow, 2002).

Provincial governments also provide and subsidize a host of health and health care services beyond those defined as universally insured services under the Canada Health Act. These include provincial prescription drug plans that fill in some of the gaps left by employment-based private health insurance provided as part of employment benefit packages for Canadians working in the public sector and for larger employers in the private sector. Provincial governments also subsidize to a considerable extent long-term care, including facility-based nursing home care and home care. Some dental and vision care services are also provided to residents who receive provincial social assistance – welfare, as it is known in most countries. These services and subsidies now constitute close to 40 per cent of provincial spending on health care (CIHI, 2011a).

Until the early 1990s, provincial governments were largely passive payers. They paid health providers (e.g., hospitals, doctors, dentists) to provide health services, or subsidized individuals (e.g., residents of long-term care facilities) to obtain access to health services. In response to a near-crisis in public finance caused by an economic downturn and accumulated debt payments, as well as

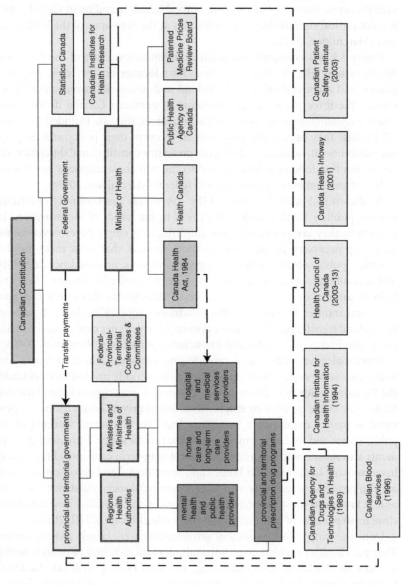

Figure 3.2 Federal-provincial organization of the Canadian health system

the desire to better coordinate and integrate the many services they funded, most provincial governments began to manage their systems through arm's-length public bodies known as regional health authorities (RHAs). While there were other reasons for this organizational reform, including the objectives of bringing the administration of health services closer to populations and allocating a larger share of public resources to public health and preventative care, the debt crisis was the most immediate pressure that produced the spate of regionalization reforms in the 1990s (Marchildon, 2006, 2016).

Through provincial laws, RHAs have a mandate to coordinate the delivery of a broad range of health and health care services to populations within their geographic borders. The two exceptions are provincial prescription drug coverage plans, which continue to be operated by provincial health ministries, and physician services, which operate largely on contracts between health ministries and provincial medical associations (Lewis & Kouri, 2004). This produces an odd result in that doctors who are working in RHA facilities are paid by provincial governments rather than RHAs. More importantly, when it comes to primary care, RHAs have limited responsibilities relative to provincial ministries.

There are some differences among provinces in terms of the RHA budget allocation formulas used by provincial governments and the extent of the services that RHAs are expected to administer. However, these are minor differences compared to the issue of whether RHAs have a mandate to both purchase and provide services or simply to purchase services. In nine provinces, RHAs can choose whether to deliver the services directly through their own organizations or to do so through contracted providers. In one province, Ontario, RHAs – known as local health integration networks – can only purchase (i.e., pay for) services from other providers, and use the tools of contract management and performance indicators to obtain the same objectives as RHAs in the rest of Canada (Marchildon, 2013a).

This introduction of a new managerial mechanism was both decentralizing and centralizing. It was decentralizing in that provincial governments transferred a majority of their health budgets – roughly two-thirds on average – to the RHAs. It was centralizing in that governance and ownership of individual hospitals and other health facilities moved from community-based organizations and local governments up to the RHAs, thereby putting more managerial control in the hands of provincial ministries of health (Axelsson, Marchildon, & Repullo-Labrador, 2007; Marchildon, 2006).

Employing the standard classification of decentralization, this change involved a weaker form of decentralization, somewhere between deconcentration and delegation but far from full-fledged devolution (Rondinelli, 1981; Rondinelli, Nellis, & Chapman, 1984). RHAs were, in effect, special operating agencies of the provincial government. It is interesting to note the extent to which provincial governments simply bypassed democratically elected governments at the local and municipal levels when they introduced RHAs, and the geographical boundaries, even in the first iteration, often exceeded those of local governments by a considerable margin. Although they enjoy greater freedom from provincial bureaucratic rules in terms of human resource management and salaries, RHAs do not have the ability to raise revenues and, in most cases, are without a democratic mandate in terms of the election of board members. RHAs were entirely dependent on provincial transfers for their expenditures and, although given the responsibility to allocate their own operating budgets, were subject to provincial priority setting and to provincial decisions concerning major capital investments such as hospital construction.

To cope with the inevitable policy overlaps and interdependencies, the provincial and federal ministers of health and their civil servants work through a thick network of intergovernmental councils, working groups, and advisory committees which report to the Conference of Federal/Provincial/Territorial (F/P/T) Deputy Minister of Health (the most senior civil servant in the ministry), which in turn report to the Conference of F/P/T Ministers of Health. The Conference of F/P/T Ministers of Health is co-chaired by the federal minister and a provincial minister selected on a rotating basis, mirrored by an identical arrangement for the Conference of F/P/T Deputy Ministers of Health. In order to conduct their work in priority areas of concern, the ministers and their chief officials have established, reorganized, and disbanded various advisory groups and task forces over time, including those dealing with health delivery and human resources, information and emerging technologies, population health, health security, and governance and accountability. These intergovernmental practices date back to the Dominion Council of Health of the 1950s, although with one important change reflecting the overall decentralization of the Canadian federation. While the federal minister of health chaired the Dominion Council of Health and set the agenda for intergovernmental meetings, the Conference of F/P/T Ministers of Health has been co-chaired and the agenda co-managed between the federal and the provincial government since the 1970s (Marchildon, 2013a).

Policy interdependencies and complexities grew over time, overtaxing the capacity of the intergovernmental conference system. As a consequence, F/P/T ministers and deputy ministers of health established an alphabet soup of arm's-length, special-purpose intergovernmental agencies to support longer-term work in areas they deemed a priority to offset the fragmentation caused by a highly decentralized health system. Consistent with the asymmetrical nature of the Canadian federation, some provinces, most notably Québec, have chosen not to join some of these organizations. Shown in Figure 3.2, these F/P/T special operating agencies include the Canadian Agency for Drugs and Technologies in Health (CADTH), the Canadian Institute for Health Information, Canada Health Infoway, the Canadian Patient Safety Institute (CPSI), and, until 2014 when its funding from the federal government ceased, the Health Council of Canada (Marchildon, 2015). All are relatively recent innovations, a voluntary way of obtaining some of the benefits of a more nationally coordinated health system without having the federal government perform these functions directly. A number of these agencies have their head offices outside Ottawa: Canada Health Infoway in Montreal, the Health Council of Canada in Toronto, and CPSI in Edmonton.

There has also been interprovincial collaboration. All provinces, with the exception of Québec, joined together to form Canadian Blood Services (CBS) in response to a tainted blood controversy and the exit of the Canadian Red Cross from the management of blood products and services. Québec created its own blood products and services agency known as Héma-Québec (Wilson, McCrea-Logie, & Lazar, 2004). While CBS board members are nominated by provincial ministers of health, civil servants are not permitted on the board to ensure that the organization is governed at arm's length from the contributing governments.

Created in 1989, CADTH's mandate is to collect, generate, and disseminate health technology analyses of new medical technologies and pharmaceutical therapies. Since there are a number of provincial health technology assessment (HTA) organizations, CADTH coordinates the dissemination of these studies as well as its own HTAs on devices and pharmaceuticals not assessed by the provincial agencies. It should be noted that CADTH's recommendations are only advisory in nature; it remains the prerogative of a provincial government to decide whether to introduce a given medical technology in its health system or to add a particular pharmaceutical to its prescription drug plan. CADTH is funded by Health Canada and by provincial and territorial governments in proportion to population. Québec is not a member and conducts its own Institute national d'excellence en santé et en services sociaux (INESSS).

Established in 1994, CIHI was an organizational response to the desire of federal and, in particular, provincial governments – again initially with the exception of Québec – for a nationally coordinated approach to gathering and analysing financial, administrative, and health service data generated by provincial governments and organizations. CIHI maintains twenty-seven databases and clinical registries, including those for health expenditures, physicians, hospital morbidity, discharge abstracts, prescription drug utilization, and information systems. CIHI also provides analyses of health data to facilitate evidence-based decision-making among partner governments. Despite the fact that provincial governments and their agencies are the main beneficiaries of CIHI, the federal government pays for 80 per cent of CIHI's operating expenses, leaving the remaining 20 per cent to be picked up by the provinces.

Since its establishment in 2001, Canada Health Infoway has been using its funding to accelerate the development and implementation of electronic health technologies, such as electronic health and medical records, as well as electronic public health surveillance systems. Almost entirely funded by the federal government ($2.1 billion from 2001 until 2011), Health Infoway also acts as a national umbrella organization to facilitate the interoperability of existing provincial electronic health information initiatives. Health Infoway includes all provincial governments, including (unusually) the government of Québec, as subscribing members.

Established in 2003, CPSI was mandated to exercise a leadership role in building a culture of patient safety and quality improvement, promoting best practices and advising governments and organizations on state-of-the-art strategies to improve patient safety. CPSI is funded principally by the federal government, but it is governed by a board made up of individuals appointed by all participating governments, giving the provinces a major voice in the direction of the organization.

The Health Council of Canada was formed in 2003 by the federal government and eight provinces but ceased operating in 2014 when a Conservative federal government, which viewed health care as the responsibility of individual provincial governments, refused to extend federal funding. The mandate of the Health Council was to monitor and report on the implementation of commitments made in federal-provincial health accords, as well as provide pan-Canadian studies on the progress made in priority reforms such as primary health care and pharmaceutical coverage policies. Alberta and Québec turned down membership, although Alberta, with a change in premier and government outlook, reversed its position and joined in 2012. The board of the Health Council of Canada was chaired by an individual nominated by consensus of the participating ministers of health, and all other board members were nominated by participating governments. With the Health Council's demise, it is unclear what will take its place, if anything (Marchildon, 2015).

Assessing Health System Decentralization and Centralization

While a description of the structural features of the Canadian federation provides the essential context for understanding the nature of decentralization in the health system, it is not sufficient to make any determinations about the degree to which the health system is either decentralized or centralized. In the next section, though, decision space analysis, first developed by Bossert (1998), is applied to various discrete aspects of publicly financed health care in Canada. This is followed by a comparison of provincial and federal health system capacity and the impact of federal transfers on provincial capacity in particular. Finally, and most speculatively, some assessment is made of the culture of federalism as it applies to the health sector. According to Mitchell and Bossert (2010), accountability, in terms of both federal-provincial accountability and accountability to citizens, is a key dimension linking governance and health system performance. As such, some discussion of accountability will accompany this analysis when directly relevant.

Gauging Decision Space in the Canada Health System

Using the decision space methodology, judgments (based on the secondary and grey literature and on the author's past experiences as an advisor and senior government official in federal-provincial negotiations) are made concerning the relative level (narrow, moderate, or broad) of authority in exercising federal and provincial government health system responsibilities. These judgments will be grouped into sectors: governance and legislative ability; rules for citizen access to health coverage and services; human resource management; choice of organizational form for coverage and delivery; and financing methods.

First, the decision space between the federal and provincial governments is examined. However, it needs to be emphasized that, unlike unitary countries such as Colombia, which Bossert (1998) used as his chief illustration of the decision space methodology, Canada's two orders of government are constitutionally sovereign in their respective areas of jurisdiction. Therefore, decision space cannot be seen as the "range of effective choice that is *allowed* by the central authorities to be utilized by local authorities" (Bossert, 1998, p. 1518, emphasis added). Instead, it is the range of effective choice actually exercised, and enabled under the constitution, by the provinces. Moreover, when it comes to health care, since the primary jurisdiction rests with the provinces (as discussed above), the provinces historically had to allow the federal government to play a role, rather than the other way around. It did this using the leverage of its own revenues by making fiscal transfers to the provinces to achieve national health system objectives that it negotiated with the provinces. This "spending power" is a policy tool used by central governments in all federations (Watts, 2008).

The federal government's involvement in provincial health care occurred in stages. The first involved the negotiations between 1955 and 1957 that led to a federal-provincial agreement in which the federal government encouraged those provinces that had not yet implemented universal hospital insurance to do so based on a set of national conditions; in return the federal government shared 50 per cent of the costs of the new program through a federal transfer to all eligible provincial governments. Between 1958 and 1961, all provincial governments implemented universal, single-payer hospital insurance with the federal conditions for shared-cost financing set out in federal law, the Hospital Insurance and Diagnostic Services Act (1957), and in bilateral agreements between Ottawa and individual provinces (Marchildon, 2012; Taylor, 1987).

The second stage required another round of federal-provincial negotiations from 1965 until 1967; between 1968 and 1971, all provincial governments implemented universal, single-payer insurance for medical care. Again, the federal government's conditions – the national principles of public administration, comprehensiveness (in terms of physician services), universality, and portability – were set out in the Medical Care Act (1966), passed by the Parliament of Canada. However, unlike the case of universal hospital insurance, the federal government did not require bilateral agreements from each province, largely in response to Québec's refusal to accept such an agreement with its associated audits and sanctions. Now, the provinces simply had to act in general conformity to the four principles enshrined in the federal law (Bryden, 2012). Eighteen years later, the Canada Health Act (1984) replaced both laws, eliminating the bilateral agreements for hospital insurance and establishing a system in which provincial governments provided an annual report on their conformity to the law's principles (Marchildon, 2014; Taylor, 1987).

The historical context is essential to understanding the decision space of the provinces, as illustrated by function in Table 3.1. The only real constraint on provincial autonomy in the administration and delivery of publicly funded health care stems from the principles or "criteria" stipulated in the Canada Health Act. Moreover, Table 3.1 is limited to hospital and physician services, since these are the only services governed by the Canada Health Act. There are effectively no limits on almost all other health services funded or subsidized by provincial governments, even including prescription drug plans, other than respecting national patent law and drug safety regulations (Marchildon, 2013a).

In terms of governance, the Canada Health Act requires provincial governments to have a publicly administered insurance scheme for hospital and physician services, but the act does not stipulate how this is to be done. As long as provincial governments are accountable for the management of coverage to their residents through their respective legislative assemblies, this is sufficient. They can administer the coverage directly through their respective ministries of health (as all provinces do now) or through arm's-length commissions (as many did historically), but they cannot contract out these functions to private insurers, for example. While the federal criteria of public administration is not explicit as to whether provincial governments must be the sole insurer, in fact all provincial governments act as single payers, and six provincial governments legally prohibit the sale of insurance by private carriers for medically necessary hospital and physician services (Flood & Archibald, 2001; Marchildon, 2005). No other federal governance requirements or limits are placed on provincial governments, and there is considerable diversity in terms of the governance, size, number, and composition of publicly funded health organizations in the provinces, and where there are similarities, these are not due to any federal requirement or standard (Marchildon, 2013b).

Although fiscally autonomous relative to other federal subnational states, provincial governments are accustomed to receiving substantial federal transfers for provincial health expenditures. Until the late 1970s when a block transfer was introduced, these federal transfers were for provincial spending on medically necessary hospital and physician services alone. These constituted 50 per cent of total provincial spending on such universally insured services. However, with the introduction of the Established Programs Financing block transfer, the federal government made a permanent tax transfer, or one-half of the block transfer, and continued to transfer the other half in cash to the provinces annually. With the cash transfer's growth now limited to the rate of overall economic growth, the provinces could spend the block transfer for any health service. Although this block transfer has gone through three iterations since the 1970s, the Canada Health and Social Transfer (1995–2003) and the Canada Health Transfer (2004–14 and 2015–present), there were no fundamental changes to the design (Marchildon & Mou, 2013, 2014). In other words, the block transfer marked a permanent change from federal earmarking to provincial autonomy in setting health spending priorities (Coyte & Landon, 1990).

The only additional earmarking has involved marginal transfers provided in addition to the regular block transfer, including those that accompanied First Ministers' agreements on health in 2000, 2003, and 2004. However, the objectives set by First Ministers often lacked specificity, and there was never really any threat that the federal government would refuse or claw back the transfers from provincial governments. For this reason, the federal limits placed on these provincial expenditure allocations were minimal (see Table 3.1).

While the cash portion of the Canada Health Transfer amounts to roughly 25–30 per cent of provincial hospital and physician expenditures, it constitutes less than 20 per cent of total provincial government expenditures on health care (Marchildon & Mou, 2014). Whether federal transfers are assessed in terms of their contribution to hospital and physician services alone (as was once

Table 3.1 Provincial decision space for Canada Health Act (universally insured hospital and physician) services

Function	Indicator	Range of Choice		
		Narrow	Moderate	Wide
Financing				
Sources of revenue	Federal transfers as % of total hospital and physician spending		Receive 25–30% from federal government	
Expenditure allocation	% of provincial spending explicitly earmarked by federal government			Earmarking very marginal and limited oversight
User fees	Extent to which provincial governments can raise funds through user fees for "insured" services		User fees subject to federal transfer withdrawals	
Service organization and delivery				
Required programs	Rules on what services must be delivered		Determination of what is included as medically necessary	
Payment mechanisms	Rules on payments to hospitals and physicians			No limits
Hospital autonomy	Choice of how hospitals governed, organized, and paid			No limits
Physician autonomy	Choice of how physicians governed, organized, and paid			No limits

Human resources		
Salaries	Choice of salary range	No limits
Contracting	Contracting non-permanent staff	No limits
Civil service	Hiring and firing	No limits
Access rules		
Targeting	Extent to which subpopulations or services can be targeted	"Insured" services must be provided to all residents
Portability	Extent to which reciprocal billing upheld by provinces for residents and non-residents	Law stipulates reciprocal billing among provinces but limited federal enforcement for medical services
Governance rules		
Insurance structure	Degree of direction on insurance structure	Publicly administered
Other administration	Federal rules limiting size, number of, composition of provincial health organizations	No limits

the practice) or their contribution to all provincial health services (which has become the practice since the 1970s), it has a moderate impact on provincial governments. The health transfer's potential withdrawal, while not crippling provincial governments, might not prevent higher-income provinces from continuing their universal coverage policies but might prevent lower-income provinces from delivering a full range of hospital and physicians services at no cost to residents. As for the permanent tax transfer that was part of the Established Programs Financing agreement, it can have no real effect on provincial behaviour. A tax transfer, once given, is almost impossible to take back and therefore has had no continuing impact on the provinces. Indeed, provincial governments consistently reject efforts by the federal government to continue to count the value of the tax transfer as part of its contribution to the provinces for health funding (Lazar & St-Hilaire, 2004; Romanow, 2002).

The one area in which federal rules have had a major impact on provincial practice involves the discretion, or lack thereof, of provincial governments and their delegated health agencies and providers to charge fees for medically necessary hospital and physician services. When universal hospital and medical care coverage was first implemented, the federal government expected provincial programs to offer the services without financial barriers, but after the first block transfer was introduced, a few provincial governments looked the other way as some hospitals and physicians charged additional fees to patients. To stop this practice, the federal government introduced a fifth principle – *accessibility* – when it introduced the Canada Health Act in 1984, along with a provision that made it mandatory for Ottawa to reduce its cash transfer, dollar for dollar, to any province that permitted these fees. A strong positive incentive was also introduced in 1984: any province that eliminated all user fees within a period of three years would have its original deductions refunded.

Since that time, provincial governments have been relatively vigilant in ensuring that hospital and doctors do not impose patient fees at the point of service, in part because of the threat of federal intervention, but more likely because of the negative publicity associated with an alleged "infraction," as the amount of money involved is small and some provinces could easily afford the deductions. There have in fact been very few (identified) violations of the accessibility criteria, the only principle where transfer deductions are required – for the four other Canada Health Act principles, both the quantum and the decision to act are within the federal cabinet's discretion. Although the federal government has threatened to use this policy tool on a handful of occasions since 1984, no province has been assessed an actual deduction for provincial infringement of the other four principles (Marchildon, 2014).

The Canada Health Act is clear on access rules. In order to receive federal health transfers, provincial governments are required to provide medically necessary hospital and physician services to all residents on the same terms and conditions. This is the definition of *universality* in the federal law, and any jurisdiction choosing to provide coverage on a categorical (e.g., income or age) basis would have to forgo its share of the Canada Health Transfer. At the same time, provincial governments are required to reimburse other jurisdictions for any hospital and medical services their residents may require while visiting other provinces or territories, as well as during the first three months after a resident moves to another province (and all provincial governments must provide universal coverage once an individual has been a resident for three months). This is known as the *portability* principle. However, due to extremely lax enforcement on the federal government's part, the portability principle began to unravel almost two decades ago, when the Government of Québec refused to reimburse the Government of Ontario for medical services at the higher Ontario tariff. Ontario retaliated by requiring Québec residents to pay up front for any medical services received in Ontario. This has been followed by tit-for-tat between Québec and other provinces as well. However, since portability continues to be respected for hospital services throughout Canada, this has been assessed as a moderate decision space for provinces (Marchildon, 2013b).

Human resource rules are not an issue for the provinces because labour management and professional organization issues lie firmly within provincial jurisdiction. As a consequence, the federal government does not attempt to regulate provincial human resource policies and norms. Any restrictions are self-imposed by provincial governments.

Similarly, the federal government has no constitutional standing to set standards or impose policies on the way in which provincial governments organize and deliver health services. There is one possible exception. If you define service organization and delivery to include the definition of the package of services offered, then provincial governments face one requirement: they must provide hospital and physician services deemed medically necessary. It is interesting to note that neither the federal nor the provincial governments have a list of what they consider medically necessary services. By federal-provincial agreement and custom, both orders of government have left this determination in the hands of physicians.

In reality, what is determined as medically necessary has been subject to confidential negotiations between the doctors' self-regulatory bodies, which operate on a provincial basis (for constitutional reasons), and provincial health ministries (Flood, Stabile, & Tuohy, 2006). Perhaps surprisingly, the list of universally insured services is remarkably similar across the country, but this need not continue to be the case. Since the determination of what constitutes medical necessity is a joint private-public decision by doctors and ministries of health at the provincial level, it might be interpreted as an area of broad decision space for provincial governments. However, future federal administrations might react negatively if a provincial government, acting in concert with the provincial college of physicians, decided to delist (not cover) a number of hospital and physician services that had traditionally been included as insured services. Given this possibility – and the knowledge of this by provincial governments – it has been assessed as a moderate, rather than broad, decision space for provinces.

Health System Capacity of Provincial Governments

As illustrated in Table 3.1, provincial governments have broad decision space authority in a majority of functional areas of health care. However, we also need to know the capacity of provincial governments to exercise their decision-making authority. This requires some generalization across provinces, a challenge given differences in relative income level and population size, both of which can have an impact on fiscal and administrative capacity.

Canadian provinces have considerable taxation authority relative to other subnational states. In effect, they have access to almost all the forms of direct and indirect taxation of the federal government, one of the reasons that Canada scores so high on Requejo's (2010) fiscal decentralization index. Of course, provinces with smaller populations, less economic diversification, and lower corporate density have shallower tax bases than larger and more economically diversified provinces. As a consequence, own-source provincial taxation capacity does vary across the provinces.

Since the 1950s, the federal government has addressed this issue through a tax redistribution program called Equalization. The purpose of Equalization is to enable less prosperous provincial governments to provide their residents with public services that are reasonably comparable to those in other provinces, at reasonably comparable levels of taxation. In 1982, Equalization became part of the Canadian constitution and, as a consequence, would be almost impossible for the federal government to dismantle (Bryden, 2014).

Given that provincial spending on health care has absorbed almost 40 per cent of the total program spending (less debt charges) by provincial governments since 2005 (CIHI, 2011b), Equalization has been an important supplement to the Canada Health Transfer in allowing less wealthy provincial governments the fiscal capacity to provide expensive programs such as Medicare (MacNevin, 2004). For provinces such as New Brunswick, Nova Scotia, Prince Edward

Island, and (at least before its very recent offshore oil boom) Newfoundland and Labrador, Equalization has contributed more to their respective treasuries than the Canada Health Transfer. Equalization is an unconditional transfer that flows into the general revenue funds of provincial governments; therefore, they can allocate the proceeds in any way they see fit. It should be noted, however, that the Canada Health Transfer also flows into the general revenue funds and therefore is only notionally earmarked to health expenditures, making it almost impossible for anyone to follow the money after it is transferred. However, since provincial health spending has grown faster than most other government program expenditures since the 1950s, it would be hard to argue that the transfers have been diverted to purposes other than health care.

In summary, provincial governments have extensive powers of taxation that are used to raise revenues for health care expenditures. This means that the potential fiscal capacity of provincial governments, in general, is high. And Equalization (in addition to the Canada Health Transfer) ensures that less wealthy provinces have the actual fiscal capacity to provide residents with access to publicly funded health services that are on par with wealthier provinces.

In contrast to fiscal capacity, which can be measured, administrative capacity is much more difficult to evaluate. The conventional wisdom is that the federal government excels in terms of its administrative capacity in taxation and regulation but is weaker than provincial governments in terms of program and service delivery. While there is little rigorous evidence to support this assertion, it is based on two propositions. The first is that, unlike the provinces, the federal government is too distant from the people it serves, and therefore less able to tailor its programs and services to the varying needs of citizens in a diverse country. The second proposition is that because of the extensive constitutional responsibilities of the provinces, the federal government actually has considerably less administrative experience than provincial governments in delivering services and is therefore not as effective at doing so.

It is also accurate to say that, over the past half century, provincial governments have gained extensive experience in health system stewardship, first as administrators of single-payer coverage systems for hospital and medical care services and subsequently as managers of health systems (Marchildon & Lockhart, 2012). However, provincial health system administrative capacity has not been compared to the health system capacity of subnational states in other federations. Nor have provinces been compared rigorously to each other. No doubt, there are differences among the provinces in terms of the critical mass of skilled and knowledgeable individuals available to perform critical health system tasks, and the differences in population size among the provinces may produce such differences.

At one extreme is Ontario, with a population of almost 13 million (38 per cent of the country's population) – the size of a number of European countries – and at the other is Prince Edward Island with its 140,000 residents. Nonetheless, while sheer population size can have an impact on the pool of qualified candidates available for health ministry and related health organization positions, there is likely enough mobility within Canada to ensure that provincial population size has not been determinative of capacity. Moreover, smaller provincial governments – Saskatchewan, with a population hovering around the 1 million mark, providing the most salient historical example – have demonstrated deep capacity and great organizational innovation in health policy and administration in the postwar era despite smaller populations (Houston, 2002; Ostry, 2006; Taylor, 1987).

Federalism Culture

The earlier discussion concerning intergovernmental activities could lead to the conclusion that there is a vibrant culture of federalism when it comes to health care in Canada. To some extent, this is true. Ministers of health and their most senior officials devote a "sizeable" share of their time to intergovernmental activities and processes.[1] However, it is a truncated culture, focused solely on executive federalism, in contrast to a number of other federations where there is the possibility of decision-making through legislative federalism, such as the Senate in Australia. In Canada, the institutions of executive federalism have produced a culture in which complete consensus is required before decisions can be made and implemented. There are no majority decision rules and almost all discussions are held in camera (O'Reilly, 2001).

Thus, federal-provincial health system decisions are painstakingly slow and must be at a very high level of generality in order to gain approval. This limits the possibility of major health reform decisions being taken at a pan-Canadian level and makes it more likely for major innovations to occur by provincial governments acting alone – perhaps providing a model which can be adopted in the rest of the country, either through imitation or through the encouragement of the federal government using its spending power.

At the same time, federal-provincial ministers of health and their senior bureaucrats have responded to these constraints by creating specialized intergovernmental operating agencies. These arm's-length agencies have more

---

1 In my own governmental experience, I have seen it absorb up to 50 per cent of the time of a provincial deputy minister of health.

autonomy in decision-making and have proved an innovative response to this constrained environment. These agencies share a similar history. With limited administrative capacity in their first years, most strain to achieve their objectives. However, with time and experience, most eventually find their niche and become a welcome part of the health system landscape. A few, such as the Health Council of Canada, get dismantled if they prove a threat to the funding governments, while others, such as the Canadian Institute for Health Information, have become a key part of federal and provincial government efforts at improving health system performance (Marchildon, 2015).

Federal and provincial governments have both had to adjust to a relatively new player at the intergovernmental table, one which has been outside the system of executive federalism. The courts have become more active in defining the rules under which the federal government and the provinces administer publicly funded health services. Although the courts have not been particularly active in reinterpreting the division of powers between the two orders of government, the Supreme Court of Canada has issued major judgments involving the Charter of Rights and Freedoms, which became part of the constitution in 1982. One of the most publicized cases involved the issue of whether the Québec government's prohibition of private health insurance of medically necessary hospital and medical services contravened the "right to life, liberty and security of the person." The Supreme Court of Canada decided that if the wait lists for elective surgery were not shortened in the province, then the Québec government would have to allow individuals to purchase private health insurance. The provincial government responded by providing care guarantees in terms of wait times and allowing individuals to purchase private health insurance for selected interventions, such as hip and knee replacements (Flood, 2007; Flood, Roach, & Sossin, 2005).

Trends and Conclusion

Over the past half century, there has been one consistent long-term trend. The federal government has retreated from its highly activist role in universal hospital insurance in the late 1950s to one that has impinged less and less on provincial authority and decision space in health care (Marchildon, 2013b). When it introduced cost-sharing for universal medical care services in the second half of the 1960s, the federal government eliminated the requirement for detailed federal-provincial agreements and concomitant audits.

When the federal government replaced cost-sharing with block transfers through Established Programs Financing in the 1970s, it eliminated transfers earmarked for medically necessary hospital and physician services. Although the passage of the Canada Health Act marked an attempt to clarify and more effectively enforce federal conditionality, the federal government's lack of enforcement of the law since at least the mid-1990s has translated into a more laissez-faire stance. At the end of 2011, when the federal government unilaterally announced changes to the Canada Health Transfer, it also made it clear that it viewed health care as a provincial responsibility and would not be seeking to establish pan-Canadian direction through intergovernmental negotiation (Marchildon & Mou, 2013).

For their part, provincial governments have reiterated their view that health care is a provincial jurisdiction, implying that it is exclusively provincial. Some provinces, in particular Québec and Alberta, have historically demanded less federal conditionality on health transfers. While federal administrations have historically disputed the claim of exclusive provincial jurisdiction, the federal government, led by Conservative prime minister Stephen Harper from 2006 until 2015, seemed to support this claim (Marchildon, 2013b). It is too early to tell whether the federal administration under Liberal prime minister Justin Trudeau will change this trajectory.

While there is a long-term trend to decentralization in terms of the two constitutionally recognized orders of governments, there has been a contrary trend to centralization at the provincial level. Although it is exceedingly difficult to generalize across provinces because each provincial government varies in its approach to regionalization, Table 3.2 describes the decision space allocated by provincial governments to RHAs in the key functional areas. What is interesting is less the limited nature of the decision-making authority within the discretion of RHAs than the fact that provincial changes in the last few years have tended to reduce this discretion, including through using key indicators as part of a more intensive system of performance measurement, as is being done by the local health integration networks (LHINs) in Ontario. Some provincial governments, most notably Alberta (2008) and Manitoba (2012), have significantly reduced the number of RHAs in order to eliminate what they considered excessive executive compensation for chief executive officers and reduced the total number of health system executives in the provincial health system. Still others, such as British Columbia and Saskatchewan, have introduced single, provincialwide organizations to manage back-office functions for RHAs such as payroll, procurement, laundry, food services, and information management systems.

Given the fact that Canada is one of the most decentralized federations in the world, it is hardly surprising that the country also has a relatively decentralized health sector. What may be more surprising is the growing trend towards decentralization from the federal to the provincial governments. Again, however, this may be simply reflective of the trend towards fiscal and political

Table 3.2 Regional health authority (RHA) decision space for Canada Health Act for the administration and delivery of publicly funded health services delegated by provincial health ministries

Function	Indicator	Range of Choice		
		Narrow	Moderate	Wide
Financing				
Source of revenue	Provincial funding as a % of RHA spending	Almost 100% of revenues from provincial governments		
Expenditure allocation	% of spending explicitly earmarked by provincial government		Some latitude in terms of operating expenditures but capital spending set by provincial government	
Fees	Extent to which RHA can raise revenues through fees for services	Policies and tariffs set by provincial government		
Procurement	Extent to which RHA can set its own procurement rules		Mixture of RHA discretion and provincial policies and rules	
Service organization and delivery				
Required programs	Rules on what services must be delivered	Set by provincial government		
Hospital autonomy	Choice of how hospitals governed, organized, and paid		Mixture of RHA and provincial decision	
Physician autonomy	Choice of how physicians governed, organized, and paid	Almost entirely set by provincial government in direct negotiation with provincial medical association		

(Continued)

Table 3.2 Regional health authority (RHA) decision space for Canada Health Act for the administration and delivery of publicly funded health services delegated by provincial health ministries (Continued)

Function	Indicator	Range of Choice		
		Narrow	Moderate	Wide
Human resources				
Salaries	Choice of salary range		Increasing limits due to provincial concerns about RHA executive compensation	Few provincial limits
Contracting	Contracting non-permanent staff			Few provincial limits
Employees	Hiring and firing	Constrained by provincial collective bargaining with major provider groups such as nurses		
Access rules				
Targeting	Extent to which subpopulations or services can be targeted	"Insured" services must be provided to all residents	Although "insured" services must be provided to all, targeting of other services permitted	
Population served	Extent to which RHA can determine whether it should provide services to individuals not resident within RHA boundaries	Provincial government sets policy in terms of service		
Governance rules				
Board appointment	Degree to which board members elected by public or appointed by existing board members	Board members appointed by ministries of health	Some or all board members elected	
Mandate	Degree to which RHA can set own mandate, or if provincially set, the flexibility of mandate		Set by provincial law in very general terms	

decentralization, a common feature among multinational federations with potentially secessionist subnational states, as is the case of Québec in Canada. The important question concerns the effectiveness of governments in managing health care in such a centralized system, and in Canada there appear to have been two responses.

The first is the creation of a number of special-purpose intergovernmental agencies by the federal and provincial governments to deal with the inevitable policy interdependencies. Of particular note is the adjustment by Ottawa to this relatively new form of organization building and, even more, its willingness to pay the lion's share of the operations of agencies despite the fact that their benefits flow mainly to provincial governments.

The second is the trend within provincial governments to exercise increasing managerial control over their respective health systems, first through regionalization and then through an increasing tendency to greater centralization after the first phase of regionalization. The end result is, from the perspective of local government and the RHAs, highly centralized control by provincial ministries of health and (perhaps) too-limited local input.

REFERENCES

Axelsson, R., Marchildon, G.P., & Repullo-Labrador, J.R. (2007). Effects of decentralization on managerial dimensions of health systems. In R.B. Saltman, V. Bankauskaite, & K. Vrangbæk (Eds.), *Decentralization in health care* (pp. 141–66). Maidenhead, NY: Open University Press & McGraw-Hill.

Bossert, T. (1998). Analyzing the decentralization of health systems in developing countries: Decision space, innovation and performance. *Social Science & Medicine, 47*(10), 1513–27. https://doi.org/10.1016/S0277-9536(98)00234-2

Braën, A. (2004). Health and the distribution of powers in Canada. In T. McIntosh, P.G. Forest, & G.P. Marchildon (Eds.), *The governance of health care in Canada* (pp. 25–49). Toronto, ON: University of Toronto Press. https://doi.org /10.3138/9781442681392-004

Bryden, P.E. (2012). The Liberal Party and the achievement of national Medicare. In G.P. Marchildon (Ed.), *Making Medicare: New perspectives on the history of Medicare in Canada* (pp. 71–88). Toronto, ON: University of Toronto Press.

Bryden, P.E. (2014). "Pooling our resources": Equalization and the origins of regional universality, 1937–1957. *Canadian Public Administration, 57*(3), 401–18. https:// doi.org/10.1111/capa.12077

CIHI. (2011a). *National health expenditures trends, 1975 to 2011*. Ottawa, ON: Canadian Institute for Health Information.

CIHI. (2011b). *Health care cost drivers: The facts*. Ottawa, ON: Canadian Institute for Health Information.

Coyte, P.C., & Landon, S. (1990). Cost-sharing and block-funding in a federal system: A demand systems approach. *Canadian Journal of Economics/Revue Canadienne d'Economique, 23*(4), 817–38. https://doi.org/10.2307/135564

Fierlbeck, K., & Palley, H.A. (2015). Canada. In K. Fierlbeck & H.A. Palley (Eds.), *Comparative health care federalism* (pp. 107–22). London, UK: Routledge.

Flood, C.M. (2007). Choulli's legacy for the future of Canadian health care policy. In B. Campbell & G.P. Marchildon (Eds.), *Medicare: Facts, myths, problems and promise* (pp. 256–91). Toronto, ON: James Lorimer and Company.

Flood, C.M., & Archibald, T. (2001). The illegality of private health care in Canada. *Canadian Medical Association Journal, 164*(6), 825–30.

Flood, C.M., Roach, K., & Sossin, L. (Eds.). (2005). *Access to care, access to justice: The legal debate over private health insurance in Canada*. Toronto, ON: University of Toronto Press. https://doi.org/10.3138/9781442670587

Flood, C.M., Stabile, M., & Tuohy, C. (2006). What is in and out of Medicare? Who decides. In C.M. Flood (Ed.), *What's in, what's out, how we decide* (pp. 15–41). Toronto, ON: University of Toronto Press. https://doi.org/10.3138/9781442676459-003

Houston, C.S. (2002). *Steps on the road to Medicare: Why Saskatchewan led the way*. Montreal, QC: McGill-Queen's University Press.

Lazar, H., & St-Hilaire, F. (2004). *Money, politics and health care: Reconstructing the federal-provincial partnership*. Montreal, QC: Institute for Research on Public Policy.

Lavoie, J.G. (2004). The values and challenges of separate services: First Nations in Canada. In J. Healy & M. McKee (Eds.), *Accessing healthcare: Responding to diversity* (pp. 325–49). Oxford, UK: Oxford University Press.

Leeson, H. (2004). Constitutional jurisdiction over health and health care services in Canada. In T. McIntosh, P.-G. Forest, & G.P. Marchildon (Eds.), *The governance of health care in Canada* (pp. 50–82). Toronto, ON: University of Toronto Press. https://doi.org/10.3138/9781442681392-005

Lewis, S., & Kouri, D. (2004). Regionalization: Making sense of the Canadian experience. *Healthcare Papers, 5*(1), 12–31. https://doi.org/10.12927/hcpap .2004.16847

MacNevin, A.S. (2004). *The Canadian federal-provincial equalization regime: An assessment*. Toronto, ON: Canadian Tax Foundation.

Marchildon, G.P. (1995). Fin de siècle Canada: The federal government in retreat. In P. McCarthy & E. Jones (Eds.), *Disintegration or transformation: The crisis of the state in advanced industrial societies* (pp. 133–51). New York, NY: St Martin's Press.

Marchildon, G.P. (2005). Private insurance for Medicare: Policy history and trajectory in the four western provinces. In C.M. Flood, K. Roach, & L. Sossin (Eds.),

Access to care, access to justice: The legal debate over private health insurance in Canada (pp. 429–53). Toronto, ON: University of Toronto Press. https://doi.org /10.3138/9781442670587-027

Marchildon, G.P. (2006). Regionalization and health services restricting in Saskatchewan. In C.M. Beach, R. P. Chaykowski, S. Shortt, F. St-Hilaire, & A. Sweetman (Eds.), *Health services restructuring in Canada: New evidence and new directions* (pp. 33–57). Montreal, QC: McGill-Queen's University Press.

Marchildon, G.P. (2009). Postmodern federalism and sub-state nationalism. In A. Ward & L. Ward (Eds.), *The Ashgate companion to federalism* (pp. 441–55). Farnham, UK: Ashgate Publishing.

Marchildon, G.P. (2012). Canadian Medicare: Why history matters. In G.P. Marchildon (Ed.), *Making Medicare: New perspectives on the history of Medicare in Canada* (pp. 3–18). Toronto, ON: University of Toronto Press.

Marchildon, G.P. (2013a). *Health systems in transition: Canada.* Toronto, ON: University of Toronto Press & the European Observatory on Health Systems and Policies.

Marchildon, G.P. (2013b). The future of the federal role in Canadian health care. In K. Fierlbeck & W. Lahey, (Eds.), *Health care federalism in Canada: Critical junctures and critical perspectives* (pp. 177–91). Montreal, QC: McGill-Queens University Press.

Marchildon, G.P. (2014). The three dimensions of universal Medicare in Canada. *Canadian Public Administration, 57*(3), 362–82. https://doi.org/10.1111/capa.12083

Marchildon, G.P. (2015). Academic networks for the evaluation of health system and policy performance. In A.S. Carson, J. Dixon, & K.R. Nossal (Eds.), *Toward a healthcare strategy for Canadians* (pp. 207–22). Montreal, QC: McGill-Queen's University Press for the School of Policy Studies, Queens University.

Marchildon, G.P. (2016). Regionalization: What have we learned? *Healthcare Papers, 16*(1), 8–14. https://doi.org/10.12927/hcpap.2016.24766

Marchildon, G.P., & Lockhart, W. (2012). Common trends in public stewardship of health care. In B. Rosen, A. Israeli, & S. Shortell (Eds.), *Accountability and responsibility in health care: Issues in addressing an emerging global challenge* (pp. 255–69). London, UK: World Scientific.

Marchildon, G.P., & Mou, H. (2013). The Conservative 10-Year Canada Health Transfer plan: Another fix for a generation? In C. Stoney & G.B. Doern (Eds.), *How Ottawa spends, 2013–2014: The Harper government – Mid-term blues and long range plans* (pp. 47–63). Montreal, QC: McGill-Queen's University Press.

Marchildon, G.P., & Mou, H. (2014). A needs-based allocation formula for Canada Health Transfer. *Canadian Public Policy, 40*(3), 209–23. https://doi.org/10.3138 /cpp.2013-052

Marchildon, G.P., Katapally, T.R., Beck, C.A., Abonyi, S., Episkenew, J., Pahwa, P., & Dosman, J.A. (2015). Exploring policy driven systemic inequities to differential access to care among Indigenous populations with obstructive sleep apnea.

International Journal for Equity in Health, 14(1), 148. https://doi.org/10.1186/s12939-015-0279-3

Mitchell, A., & Bossert, T.J. (2010). Decentralisation, governance and health-system performance: "Where you stand depends on where you sit." *Development Policy Review, 28*(6), 669–91. https://doi.org/10.1111/j.1467-7679.2010.00504.x

O'Reilly, P. (2001). The Federal/Provincial/Territorial health conference system. In D. Adams (Ed.), *Federalism, democracy and Canadian health policy.* Montreal, QC: McGill-Queens' University Press.

Ostry, A. (2006). *Change and continuity in Canada's health care system.* Ottawa, ON: Canadian Healthcare Association.

Requejo, F. (2010). Federalism and democracy: The case of minority nations, a federalist deficit. In M. Burgess & A. Gagnon (Eds.), *Federal democracies* (pp. 275–98). London, UK: Routledge.

Romanow, R.J. (2002). *Building on values: The future of health care in Canada: Final report of the Commission on the Future of Health Care in Canada.* Saskatoon, SK: Commission on the Future of Health Care in Canada.

Rondinelli, D.A. (1981). Government decentralization in comparative perspective: Theory and practice in developing countries. *International Review of Administrative Sciences, 47*(2), 133–45. https://doi.org/10.1177/002085238004700205

Rondinelli, D.A., Nellis, J.R., & Chapman, G.S. (1984). *Decentralization in developing countries: A review of recent experience.* Washington, DC: World Bank.

Taylor, M.G. (1987). *Health insurance and Canadian public policy: The seven decisions that created the Canadian healthcare system* (2nd ed.). Montreal, QC: McGill Queen's University Press.

Watts, R.L. (2008). *Comparing federal systems* (3rd ed.). Kingston, ON: McGill-Queen's University Press for the Institute of Intergovernmental Affairs.

Wilson, K., McCrea-Logie, J., & Lazar, H. (2004). Understanding the impact of intergovernmental relations on public health: Lessons from reform initiatives in the blood system and health surveillance. *Canadian Public Policy, 30*(2), 177–94. https://doi.org/10.2307/3552391

Chapter Four

Germany: The Increasing Centralization of the Health Care Sector

STEFAN GREß AND STEPHANIE HEINEMANN

Structural Features of the German Federal State

In contrast to other federations such as Spain, Canada, Belgium, or the United Kingdom, the Federal Republic of Germany is not a plurinational but a uninational federation.[1] Still, the degree of constitutional federalism – measured by Requejo on a 20-point scale – is rather high and on a level with plurinational federations. In contrast, Requejo found the degree of decentralization is lower than in Canada or Belgium but higher than in quasi-federal Spain and the United Kingdom (Requejo, 2010). This first view on the issues of constitutional federalism and the degree of decentralization already points to the fact that in the German federation it is the participation of the states (*Länder*) in the legislative process, rather than the delegation of powers within the executive power, that determines the degree of decentralization.

In Germany, a special brand of cooperative federalism has developed since the foundation of the German national state in 1871. Decentralization does have a very specific connotation in the context of federalism and health care in Germany. With regard to the establishment of a rather generous welfare state in general and the development of health care financing and delivery in particular, the central government and the states have come to terms at the expense of a third party (Manow, 2004). This means that health care is financed predominantly by contributions borne by employers and employees – not by state or national taxes. Moreover, responsibility and authority in the domain of health

---

1 For a theoretical and empirical distinction between these two types of federations, see Requejo (2010). Empirically, plurinational federations are characterized by a "distinct party system from that of its state-level counterpart within which at least one secessionist party is present" (Requejo, 2010, p. 277).

care is legally entrusted in semi-autonomous public entities, a specific form of decentralization known as delegation (Bossert, 1998).

Peak organizations of sickness funds (health insurers) and health care providers (physicians and hospitals) constitute these semi-autonomous public entities. They operate on a meso level, between federal and state jurisdiction (macro level) on the one hand and individual sickness funds and individual health care providers (micro level) on the other hand. These entities fulfil a number of tasks on the national level – such as defining the catalogue of benefits for all sickness funds in the country. Other entities – with the same composition of sickness funds and health care providers – perform tasks at the state (*Länder*) and local (municipal) level. For example, these bodies determine payment rates for physicians and hospitals on the *Länder* level and capacity planning for physicians on the local level. This corporatist arrangement provides a very specific arena for the more recent trend towards centralization (Greß, Gildemeister, & Wasem, 2004). An increasing role of competition – primarily among individual sickness funds – challenges the traditional balance of power between the central government and federal entities in health care and has created an impetus for greater centralization (Gerlinger, 2008).

Introduction to the German Federal System and Health System Decentralization

Central institutional characteristics of the German welfare state – social health insurance being the central part of this architecture – date back to their foundation in the late nineteenth century. In general, legislative responsibility for social policy lies with the central government. However, a strong veto power of the states (*Länder*) in the legislative process led to an organizational design of the emerging social insurance schemes which was, as noted, a meso level, neither centralized nor federalist. Finally, resistance of the *Länder* against tax-financed schemes led to financial autonomy based on contributions of affiliates and a para-fiscal status of the sickness funds. Thus, the strong reliance of the German welfare state on contributions was, to a very large extent, a political solution to a conflict between the central government and the *Länder*. Moreover, it minimized the financial involvement of both orders of government, a situation that remains the case today (Manow, 2004).

Bismarck's welfare state legislation between 1883 and 1889 had a strong pro-centralist bias. This "anti-federalist momentum" (Manow, 2005, p. 226) was exemplified by Bismarck's plan to establish a central bureaucracy responsible for the oversight of the new welfare state system (Kahlenberg & Hoffmann, 2001). This bureaucracy was supposed to be staffed by a corps of permanent civil servants. More importantly, it was supposed to be financed by taxes in order to increase

Table 4.1 Constitutional position of the federal chamber (Bundesrat) in the Imperial Constitution and in the Grundgesetz

	Imperial Constitution (1871)	Grundgesetz (1949)
Veto power (majority of Bundesrat)	Absolute veto of the Bundesrat	Absolute veto of the Bundesrat in all matters that affect state administration (50–60% of all laws) Suspending veto of the Bundesrat in all other matters
Number of states	25	16
Number of distribution of votes	58 (dominant position of Prussia: 17 votes)	68 (maximum of 6 votes for largest states)
Free mandate	Members are delegates of state governments – no free mandate	Members are delegates of state governments – no free mandate
Taxation	States receive all direct taxes – the central states receives all indirect taxes. Tax laws need the consent of the states.	Taxation is a central responsibility – extensive fiscal equalization scheme
Right to initiate legislation	Bundesrat has exclusive right to initiate legislation	Both chambers (Bundesrat and Bundestag) have the right to initiate legislation (co-legislation)

Source: Manow (2004, p. 14) and Manow (2005, p. 235)

the fiscal manoeuvrability of the central government (Manow, 2004). However, Bismarck's attempts to use the new welfare state as an instrument to increase the power of the central government met fierce resistance from the *Länder* in the federal chamber of parliament – the Bundesrat. As a result of the strong constitutional collective veto position of the *Länder*, Bismarck was forced to negotiate and abandon his centralized bureaucratic and tax-financed plan. However, the new social insurance did not follow a purely federalist design either (Manow, 2005; Stolleis, 2001, p. 265).

It is important to note that the German parliamentary system consists of two chambers. The first chamber – the Bundestag – constitutes members of the political parties as a result of general elections. The *Bundeskanzler* (chancellor or prime minister) is elected by the Bundestag only. The *Länder* send representatives to the second chamber (Bundesrat). The constitutional authority of the Bundesrat has changed over time (see Table 4.1). Today the constitution provides the Bundesrat with the right to initiate legislation and to veto all legislation that concerns administration on the state level.

While the organizational principles of the emerging Bismarck-era social insurance schemes differed among unemployment insurance, health insurance, accident insurance, and the pension scheme, these plans did not mirror the federalist structure of the German national government at that time. This is true especially for health insurance. Health insurance funds were organized either locally along company lines or by occupation as collective self-help organizations for professional groups. The spectrum of these sickness funds in terms of territorial distribution was enormous. While the majority of sickness funds were organized locally below the level of states, sickness funds for white-collar workers were organized above the level of individual states – some even at a national level.

A process of concentration and centralization has gradually reduced the number of sickness funds from as many as 20,000 in the late nineteenth century to as few as 118 in 2016. This dynamic has been driven primarily by the economic advantages of larger over smaller risk pools. Even today, smaller sickness funds may face bankruptcy due to a small number of severely ill individuals.

Bismarck's plan for a central institutional design for the welfare state was not approved in the legislature, and the same was true for his plan to finance the welfare state by tax revenue. He hoped that the responsibility of the central state for social security would legitimize tapping new sources for tax revenue (Manow, 2005). However, the financial architecture of the welfare state was again a compromise between the central state and the *Länder*. This compromise did not produce a federalist financing scheme. Instead, social contributions became the dominant source of revenue. This remains the case for health insurance in Germany. This fiscal autonomy of sickness funds increased steadily and was an important factor in the continuous growth of the welfare state in Germany until the end of the twentieth century (Manow, 2004).

German states were already sovereign bodies when the national state was established in 1871. The constitutional balance of powers was intended to establish a unified national state and to overcome fragmentation. Moreover, from the establishment of the German national state until today, centralist interventions were at least partly legitimized by the central government and accepted by the *Länder* based on a notion of uniform living conditions (Lang, 2015). Specifically, this notion legitimizes centralist interventions in the welfare sector. As Manow (2004) states, "Social legislation was *deliberately* used as an instrument of national unification and was explicitly designed to prevent a federalist fragmentation of living conditions" (p. 17; emphasis in original).

The years after the First World War and the concurrent establishment of the Weimar Republic were characterized by a trend towards centralization. This was not just an expression of a more centralist constitution, war, and economic crisis in the 1920s and early 1930s. From the very start, the German brand of federalism very much favoured national unity and legislative centralization. Still, the day-to-day administration of social health insurance remained decentralized.

Rather surprisingly, the Nazi administration's influence on social welfare was limited, with almost no change to the social insurance schemes. Although the National Socialists abolished the *Länder* in 1934, this had almost no impact on health insurance because the social insurance organizational structure was largely independent of federalism. As a consequence, the temporary ending of the federation had comparatively little consequence for the administration of social insurance (Manow, 2004).

After the liberation from the Nazi regime, the re-establishment of the *Länder* in 1947 laid the foundation for the establishment of the Federal Republic of Germany in 1949 and the assigning of responsibility for the oversight of all social insurance schemes to the states. However, the mostly consensual reassignment of responsibilities for social welfare from the *Länder* to the national level after 1949 again was legitimized by the commonly accepted idea that all Germans should enjoy a uniform definition of minimum living conditions (Lang, 2015; Manow, 2004).

The institutional setup of the welfare state in the Federal Republic of Germany essentially returned to the path set out by Bismarck. Proposals of fiscal devolution – central government would have been dependent on fiscal transfers by the *Länder* budgets – after the war were mostly motivated by tactical considerations in order to win the first federal election in 1949. However, the resistance to decentralization crossed party lines. Therefore, the widespread consensus about recentralizing the welfare state and the general sentiment against decentralizing federalism were intertwined. Moreover, this centralizing consensus was made possible by granting the *Länder* a strong veto position in all matters that affect state administration and by establishing an extensive fiscal equalization scheme (see Table 4.1). As a consequence of the latter, regional differences in tax revenue owing to differences in economic development are equalized to a large degree by a complex system of vertical transfers from the central state to the *Länder* combined with horizontal transfers from rich to poor *Länder*. Horizontal transfers (*Länderfinanzausgleich*) are based on long-term binding agreements between states (*Länder*). It is important to note that horizontal as well as vertical transfers are non-conditional, allowing the *Länder* to allocate the funds as they desire.

Constitutional Authority and Health System Organization

The West German constitution (Grundgesetz) of 1949 deliberately refrained from prescribing the institutional details of the future welfare state.[2] Instead, there is only a vague reference to Germany being a "democratic and social federal state" in Article 20 of the Grundgesetz (Manow, 2004). While the basic law does not specifically refer to health policy in general, federal law dominates in the health care sector. This dominance is based on federal jurisdiction for social health insurance, licensing for health professionals, legislation for pharmaceuticals and medical devices, and legal responsibility for the financing of current hospital costs (Article 74).

Legislation on a federal level repeatedly and extensively has made use of this constitutional dominance. Frequent health care reforms have regulated and re-regulated social health insurance, pricing, and reimbursement for pharmaceuticals and hospital financing. The German Supreme Court (Bundesverfassungsgericht) has confirmed that federal legislation in the area of social health insurance is consistent with the constitution because it considers such legislation necessary to ensure uniform minimum living conditions across the federation (BVerfG, 2005). According to Article 72 of the Grundgesetz, federal legislation can be necessary to ensure uniform minimum living conditions.

Important areas of health care legislation remain with the states – predominantly hospital planning, public health, and day-to-day administration of social health insurance (Welti, 2012). Still, most observers see a strong trend towards centralization in the area of health policy (Gerlinger, 2008). This may be true in terms of the sheer number of laws passed in numerous areas of health policy. However, the *Länder* act as a check on the dominance of the federal authority. Since most laws passed on a federal level in the area of health policy affect state administration in one way or another, the second chamber (Bundesrat) has to agree to federal legislation (Article 84 of the Grundgesetz).

The strong veto position of the *Länder* in the Bundesrat is an integral part of the German brand of federalism (Lang, 2015). Therefore, a majority of *Länder* in the Bundesrat is able to stop federally sponsored legal initiatives. It does not mean that a single *Land* or a minority in the Bundesrat is able

---

2 The Grundgesetz lost its preliminary character after reunification of Germany in 1990.

to do the same. Case studies – in particular in the health care sector – often stress that the veto power of the majority of the *Länder* in the Bundesrat has prevented more far-reaching reform measures from being enacted (Rosewitz & Webber, 1990). However, the empirical evidence for this is contested. There is little difference between legal initiatives in which the *Länder* have a strong veto position and those in which they have a weak or no veto position (Manow, 2004).

Moreover, all major health care reforms since the early 1990s have involved the *Länder* in some form even if the Bundesrat has been dominated by opposition parties. Quite often, the *Länder* participated actively in passing the laws underpinning reform. This is exemplified by the 1992 health care reform (*Gesundheitsstrukturgesetz* – GSG), which established the foundation for a system of managed competition in the German health insurance system (Reiners, 1993). This reform has been made possible by an informal grand coalition by the governing Christian Democrats and the Social Democrats. The latter were the opposition party in the first chamber (Bundestag) but dominated the Bundesrat. A similar institutional arrangement provided the basis for the 2003 reform (*GKV-Modernisierungsgesetz* – GMG) – only in the reverse order. Social Democrats and the Green Party dominated the first chamber but were forced to negotiate a compromise with Christian Democrats, who dominated the Bundesrat (Orlowski & Wasem, 2003). Even in times of the formal grand coalition between Social Democrats and Christian Democrats, representatives of *Länder* parliaments and governments are involved in negotiations. This is exemplified by the 2007 health care reform, which established the central health care fund (Pressel, 2012).

These examples underline that political deadlock situations are the exception rather than the rule. This is true even during divided governments – when there are different majorities in both chambers of Parliament (Auel, 2010). This can be explained by the fact that the "policy distance" between the major parties – Christian Democrats and Social Democrats – has never been very marked on questions of social policy (Manow, 2005, pp. 224, 225).

Assessing Health System Decentralization and Centralization

An important aspect of German federalism is the fact that the responsibility for the execution of federal law regarding social health insurance is shared by the central government and the *Länder*. In general, the constitution placed this responsibility on the *Länder* (Articles 30 and 83 Grundgesetz). However, the Grundgesetz also points out a number of important exceptions (Article 87). In the area of social health insurance, the most important exception concerns

Table 4.2 Meso-level institutions in German social health insurance

Institution	Members	Responsibilities	Regional Level	Oversight
Joint Federal Board	Peak organizations of sickness funds, hospitals, physicians	Definition of benefits package Procedures for physician planning	National	National government
Joint Federal Assessment Committee	Peak organization of sickness funds, physicians	Level of payment for outpatient physicians	National	National government
Association of Statutory Health Insurance Physicians	Elected individual physicians	Distribution of payments for physicians	State	State government
Admissions Committee	Peak organization of sickness funds, physicians	Capacity planning for physicians	Local	State government

the oversight of social health insurers. The central government is responsible for overseeing all peak organizations of social health insurers and physicians, as well as individual social health insurers operating on a national level. However, several peak organizations and even individual social health insurers operate on the state level as well. Therefore, the *Länder* are responsible for overseeing all peak organizations of social health insurers and physicians and individual social health insurers operating on a state level.

Governance Rules

Table 4.2 sums up the most important meso-level institutions in German social health insurance. The Joint Federal Board (Gemeinsamer Bundesausschuss) determines the benefits package of social health insurers and defines general guidelines for capacity planning of outpatient physicians. The members of the board are representatives of the social health insurance peak organization on the one hand and peak organizations of physicians and hospitals on the other hand. The board operates on a national level, and its guidelines are mandatory for all social health insurers and physicians and hospitals in the country. Still, central government institutions oversee the operation of the Joint Federal Board and need to acknowledge the lawfulness of its guidelines.

The Joint Federal Assessment Committee (Bewertungsausschuss) also operates on a national level. It determines the level of payment for outpatient physicians. Again, decisions are made by representatives of social health insurers on the one hand and representatives of physicians on the other hand. These decisions need to be acknowledged by central government institutions and are binding for all social health insurers and physicians in the country.

In contrast, the distribution of payments between family physicians and specialists is determined by the Association of Statutory Health Insurance Physicians (Kassenärztliche Vereinigung) on the state level. Physicians elect members of this association from their midst. The distribution of payment needs to be acknowledged by state governments and is only binding for physicians in the respective state. The Admission Committee (Zulassungsausschuss) – consisting of physician representatives and sickness funds representatives – is responsible for capacity planning on the local level. These committees are overseen by state governments as well.

Financing

The number of social health insurers (sickness funds) has declined steadily. As a consequence of ongoing concentration on the social health insurance market, health insurers increasingly operate on a national level. More than two-thirds of all health insurers operate nationally. Thus, the decision space for the *Länder* regarding the oversight of social health insurers is decreasing steadily (Gerlinger, 2008). The share of regional sickness funds declines. As a consequence, influence of the *Länder* decreases as well. Moreover, the constitutional division of responsibilities is not functional. The standards for overseeing social health insurers differ among states and between the states and the federal level. The *Länder* are closer to regional sickness funds and offer them more leeway. In contrast federal authorities are more strict regarding sickness funds operating on a national level. As a consequence, these differences distort competition between national and state health insurers operating in the same state (Ebsen, Greß, Jacobs, Szecsenyi, & Wasem, 2003).

The financing of social health insurance in Germany is based predominantly on contribution payments. Subsidies through tax financing has increased during the last decade in absolute as well as in relative terms. However, about 90 per cent of health care expenditure of social health insurance is still being raised independently of taxes (Greß, Maas, & Wasem, 2008). Thus, the core of health care financing still follows the path set out by Bismarckian legislation. However, since federal taxes now contribute to the financing of social health insurance, they also increase the decision space of the central government.

This is indicated by the fact that the minister of finance increasingly tries to influence the outcome of health care reforms.

Although the *Länder* do not have direct responsibilities for the financing of social health insurance, they oversee the calculation of the levels of individual income-dependent contributions to social health insurers' operation on a state level. Nonetheless, there is a trend towards centralization in this area (Jakubowski & Saltman, 2013). First, as noted before, the number of social health insurers operating on a state level – and the share of individuals covered by them – is declining (Gerlinger, 2008). Second, the 2007 health care reform introduced a central fund which is financed by income-dependent contributions. This fund in turn allocates risk-adjusted payments to individual social health insurers. The central fund is administrated by an autonomous federal agency which has some, though restricted, decision space to decide how to allocate resources to individual health insurers. The contribution rate for income-dependent contributions is determined by the federal government. Before 2007, the contribution rate for income-dependent contributions was determined by individual social health insurers. Today, individual health insurers are able to determine only a small nominal portion of the contribution, which is intended to stimulate price competition.

There is considerable debate whether the centralization of health care financing has been able to make health care financing more sustainable and to make price differences between social health insurers more transparent (Goepffarth, Greß, Jacobs, & Wasem, 2007). In any case, the introduction of the central fund made it easier to administer interregional transfers. Before the introduction of the central fund, state governments in more affluent states repeatedly argued against interregional transfers even though the Supreme Court has condoned these transfers as an important instrument to ensure uniform minimum living conditions in the federation. Since the introduction of the central fund, interstate transfers to social health insurers operating in less affluent states have become less visible and therefore less controversial.

By and large, individual social health insurers have very little decision space in determining their benefits package. The extent of services covered is determined in very general terms by federal legislation, while the specific content of the benefits package is then determined by decision-making bodies at the national level. The membership of these decision bodies is made up of delegates of peak organizations of social health insurers and health care providers (Greß, Niebuhr, Rothgang, & Wasem, 2005).

While the central government delegates responsibilities to these decision-making bodies, the responsibility for determining the extent of benefits package, and the oversight of these institutions, remains with the federal government (see Table 4.2). Thus, the resulting high degree of centralization can be explained by the constitutional requirement of uniform minimum living conditions in the federation. The latter also explains why services are fully portable across the country.

Service Organization and Delivery

With regard to service organization and delivery, the constitution and federal law again divides tasks between the central government and the *Länder*. This division of responsibilities is especially pronounced in the hospital sector (see Table 4.3). The market for hospitals in Germany is divided among private for-profit hospitals, private not-for-profit hospitals, and public hospitals. Private for-profit hospitals are mostly run by corporate hospital chains and have a market share of about 33 per cent. Private not-for-profit hospitals are run by religious organizations or other not-for-profit organizations. They have a market share of 36 per cent. Public hospitals, mainly owned by municipal governments, make up the remainder of the market (Statistisches Bundesamt, 2013).

Only the payment system for current costs – diagnosis-related groups or DRGs – is determined in general terms by federal law. Again, decision-making bodies on the national level determine the details of the payment system, which are binding for the whole country. In contrast, the *Länder* are responsible for hospital planning and the financing of investment costs for hospital infrastructure such as buildings and medical equipment. Therefore, the decision space for the *Länder* in these areas is considerable, reflected in sixteen different state laws for hospital planning and the considerable variation in hospital financing for investment costs (DKG, 2014).

However, the consequences flowing from the decentralization of hospital planning, as well as aspects of hospital financing, are a matter of contentious debate (Lang, 2015). States were able to build hospitals and health insurers had to pay most of the bill. Therefore, many observers argue that the high number of hospital beds per inhabitant in Germany – in many urban areas there is a pronounced and inefficient oversupply of hospital services – is a direct consequence of inefficient decentralized hospital planning (Neubauer, 2003).

Moreover, as a consequence of increasing budget deficits in the states, the *Länder* increasingly are unable – or unwilling – to come up with the financial resources for building new hospitals or even for financing necessary maintenance and improvements in existing hospitals. Between 1991 and 2011, hospital investment by the states decreased from 3.6 billion euros to 2.67 billion euros (prices not adjusted for inflation). As mentioned before, variations

Table 4.3 Decision space for *Länder* for services covered by social health insurance

Function	Indicator	Range of Choice		
		Narrow	Moderate	Wide
Financing				
Source of revenue: contributions	Autonomy of social health insurers to determine contributions	Income-dependent contribution rate determined on a federal level		Nominal premium determined by individual health insurers
Source of revenue: taxes	Federal transfers as % of total spending of social health insurers	Health insurers receive about 10% of total expenditures from federal government (not earmarked) Länder do not contribute funds Increasing fiscal constraints for Länder		
Expenditure allocation	Existence of intraregional transfers	Nationally determined risk equalization system guarantees extensive intraregional transfers (uniform living conditions)		
User fees	Extent to which health insurers can raise funds through user fees	User fees are determined on a federal level for all social health insurers		
Service organization and delivery				
Required programs	Rules on what services must be delivered	Package of benefits is determined on the federal level (uniform living conditions)		
Financing of hospitals	Financing of current costs and investment costs		Payment system for current costs determined on a federal level – some state variations	Investment costs covered by states
Hospital planning	Rules for determining the number and location of hospitals			No limits

Hospital autonomy	Choice of how hospitals are governed and organized		No limits (share of non-profit public hospitals decreasing)
Contractual autonomy of social health insurers	Selective contracting with hospitals and physicians by social health insurance	Dominance of collective contracts (autonomy is increasing)	
Human resources			
Financing of physicians	Rules on payments to physicians	Payment system determined on a federal level – some state variations	
Physician planning	Rules for determining the number and location of outpatient physicians	Procedures determined on a federal level – some regional autonomy (increasing)	
Physician autonomy	Choice of how physicians are governed and organized		No limits
Access rules			
Targeting	Extent to which subpopulations or services can be targeted	All services must be provided to all individuals insured by social health insurers	
Portability of services	Intraregional portability of services	Full portability of services	
Governance rules			
Oversight of social health insurers	Responsibility for overseeing social health insurers (with regard to financial liquidity and contracts with providers)	Federal responsibility for overseeing national social health insurers (increasing)	State responsibility for overseeing state social health insurers (declining)

between states are considerable (DKG, 2014). As a consequence, hospitals have to finance investment costs out of the budget for current costs, which in turn increases the pressure on current costs – primarily costs for human resources – and accelerates the privatization of public hospitals. Since most public hospitals are owned by municipalities and most municipal governments face even more severe budget deficits than the *Länder*, privatization is a convenient short-term solution to get rid of those public hospitals running deficits (Lang, 2015).[3] Of course, this in turn reduces the decision space of public decision makers at the local level. However, state governments oversee all hospitals in their state and are required to apply the same regulatory standards to private and public hospitals.

Although there have been numerous proposals to streamline hospital payments by shifting the responsibility for financing investment costs to social health insurers, the *Länder* have used their collective veto power in the legislative process to deflect these proposals. Naturally, the same proposals also suggested shifting the responsibility for hospital planning to social health insurers – which the *Länder* are keen to avoid.

The decision space of the states is less robust in the area of regulating outpatient physician services. Family doctors and specialists are independent private providers. Most of them – about 59 per cent – work in single-handed practices. Another 35 per cent work in group practices. The remaining 6 per cent of outpatient physicians work in health centres run either by physicians or by hospitals (KBV, 2011).

Criteria and procedures for capacity planning are determined in the most general terms in federal law. These procedures are operationalized by decision-making bodies, the members of which are made up of delegates of peak organizations of social health insurers and physicians. Only recently has federal law changed to give the states more responsibility to oversee these decision-making bodies operating at the state level – for instance, if there is an unequal regional distribution of physicians. This change of federal law was triggered by growing doubts as to the viability of the existing system in planning and preparing adequate physician services. Currently there is an oversupply of physician services in many urban municipalities at the same time there is an undersupply of physician services in many rural municipalities (Greß & Stegmüller, 2011). Remuneration of physician services is mostly determined on the federal level as well, with some variation on a state level.

---

3 Although all *Länder* have revised their constitutions in order to refrain from taking up new debt, these changes will only take effect in 2018 or later.

The Joint Federal Assessment Committee (Bewertungsausschuss) negotiates the budget available for physician payments from social health insurers. Since this same committee also determines allocation mechanisms and payment systems, there is little decision space for the *Länder* and social health insurers. The *Länder* only oversee negotiations between physicians and social health insurers to provide additional payments – such as those for taking into account regional variations of morbidity. Here, oversight means the negations follow procedural requirements. Therefore, decision space of the *Länder* in this area is rather small.

In principle, contracting between social health insurers and health care providers such as hospitals, clinics, and physicians is based on collective contracts. Individual social health insurers used to have very little decision space to contract selectively. Principally, social health insurers have to contract all health care providers determined by *Länder* hospital planning and by local capacity planning. However, for the last decade, federal law has increased the discretion of individual social health insurers to contract selectively, for example by introducing financial incentives for physicians to strengthen primary care, integrated care, and disease management programs (Greß, 2006).

This approach to strengthen competition between health insurers and health care providers delegates responsibilities away from institution on the meso level to individual health insurers and individual health care providers. However, competition among social health insurers also expands the central government's decision-making space. Competitive forces increase the trend towards concentration on the market for social health insurance. Small social health insurers need to either drop out of the market or merge with bigger competitors. However, concentration does not only imply a decreasing number of social health insurers. Another important consequence of market concentration is the increasing scale of operation. Health insurers increasingly operate nationally, which, in effect, transfers the regulatory responsibility for overseeing them to the federal level. This development in turn reduces the decision-making space for the *Länder*.

Trends and Conclusion

Trends in Health System Decentralization as a Whole

Our analysis of the decision space of the *Länder* in health care has shown that there are very few areas that show a pronounced trend towards decentralization in the last decade or so. One example concerns increasing *Länder* responsibilities for the allocation of outpatient physicians.

In contrast, federal legislation and market concentration of social health insurance have significantly decreased the discretion of the *Länder* to exert influence on health care financing and delivery. First, increasing the proportion of tax financing to contributions in the social health insurance system leads to a stronger position for the central government. The federal minister of finance has become a new player in the health policy arena, which had not been the case when contribution payments completely covered social health insurance expenditures. Second, the introduction of a central fund and the determination of a uniform contribution rate by the central government have also facilitated re-centralization. Third, market concentration and increasing the scale of operations of social health insurers have also resulted in a stronger role of the central state relative to the *Länder*. The number of social health insurers operating on a national level is increasing, which in turn results in regulatory oversight by national instead of state authorities.

This trend towards centralization resulting from federal legislation and market concentration is reinforced by rising doubts about the effectiveness of decentralized decision-making. Oversupply of hospital beds and underfinancing of investment costs of hospitals have brought into question the merits of health system decentralization. Although most of them face increasing budget deficits, so far the *Länder* are reluctant to give up their financial responsibilities for hospital financing. If social health insurers were to take over this additional financial burden, they would also demand to take over the responsibility for hospital planning. However, diverging standards for overseeing social health insurers by *Länder* authorities would only put additional pressure on federal policymakers to re-centralize responsibilities.

Conclusion

Federalism enters the health care system in Germany from three directions (Lang, 2015). First, federal laws need to be approved by the Bundesrat. Second, state governments regulate and finance large parts of hospital care. Third – and probably most importantly – the German central state traditionally delegates responsibilities to peak organization decision-making bodies in health care.

These bodies either already operate on a national level (such as decision-making bodies for determining the extent of the benefits package) or increasingly do so (such as social health insurers). Moreover, this trend towards centralization is reinforced by rising doubts about the effectiveness of decentralized decision-making. For example, the effectiveness of decentralized hospital planning by the *Länder* is rather contentious. However, it is important to note that it is not decentralized decision-making itself which is responsible for this development but increasing fiscal and political constraints (Lang, 2015).

Moreover, several recent developments – such as an increasing share of federal tax financing of social health insurance, the introduction of a central fund to allocate resources to social health insurers, and competition among social health insurers – also contribute to decreasing decision space of the *Länder*. However, these recent trends are consistent with the long-term trend of centralizing responsibilities in order to attain an important constitutional requirement, namely uniform living conditions in the German federation. As a consequence, the *Länder* increasingly have to rely on their constitutional rights of collectively participating in the legislative process via the second chamber of the German parliament (Bundesrat).

REFERENCES

Auel, K. (2010). Between *Reformstau* and *Länder* strangulation? German co-operative federalism re-considered. *Regional & Federal Studies, 20*(2), 229–49. https://doi.org /10.1080/13597561003729913

Bossert, T. (1998). Analyzing the decentralization of health systems in developing countries: Decision space, innovation and performance. *Social Science & Medicine, 47*(10), 1513–27. https://doi.org/10.1016/S0277-9536(98)00234-2

BVerfG. (2005). Beschluss des zweiten Senats des Bundesverfassungsgerichts vom 18. Juli 2005. http://www.bverfg.de/e/fs20050718_2bvf000201.html. Retrieved 8 November 2017.

DKG. (2014, January). Bestandsaufnahme zur Krankenhausplanung und Investitionsfinanzierung in den Bundesländern. Deutsche Krankenhausgesellschaft. http://www.dkgev.de/media/file/15861.RS046-14_Anlage-Bestandsaufnahme _Januar_2014.pdf. Retrieved 27 March 2014.

Ebsen, I., Greß, S., Jacobs, K., Szecsenyi, J., & Wasem, J. (2003). *Vertragswettbewerb in der gesetzlichen Krankenversicherung zur Verbesserung von Qualität und Wirtschaftlichkeit der Gesundheitsversorgung – Gutachten im Auftrag des AOK-Bundesverbandes* (vol. 13). Bonn, Germany: AOK-Bundesverband – AOK im Dialog.

Gerlinger, T. (2008). Wettbewerbsinduzierte Unitarisierung: Der Wandel der Bund-Länder-Beziehungen in der Gesundheitspolitik. In H. Scheller & J. Schmid (Eds.), *Föderale Politikgestaltung im deutschen Bundesstaat: Variable Verflechtungsmuster in Politikfeldern* (pp. 242–63). Baden-Baden, Germany: Nomos.

Goepffarth, D., Greß, S., Jacobs, K., & Wasem, J. (Eds.). (2007). *Jahrbuch Risikostrukturausgleich 2007 – Gesundheitsfonds*. St. Augustin, Germany: Asgard.

Greß, S. (2006). Regulated competition in social health insurance: A three-country comparison. *International Social Security Review, 59*(3), 27–47. https://doi.org /10.1111/j.1468-246X.2006.00246.x

Greß, S., Gildemeister, S., & Wasem, J. (2004). The social transformation of American medicine: A comparative view from Germany. *Journal of Health Politics, Policy and Law, 29*(4–5), 679–99. https://doi.org/10.1215/03616878-29-4-5-679

Greß, S., Maas, S., & Wasem, J. (2008). Social insurance versus tax financing in health care: Reflections from Germany. In C. Flood, M. Stabile, & C. Tuohy (Eds.), *Exploring social insurance: Can a dose of Europe cure Canadian health care finance?* (pp. 115–38). Kingston, ON: McGill-Queens University Press.

Greß, S., Niebuhr, D., Rothgang, H., & Wasem, J. (2005). Criteria and procedures for determining benefit packages in health care: A comparative perspective. *Health Policy (Amsterdam), 73*(1), 78–91. https://doi.org/10.1016/j.healthpol.2004.10.005

Greß, S., & Stegmüller, K. (2011). *Gesundheitliche Versorgung in Stadt und Land – Ein Zukunftskonzept*. Wiesbaden, Germany: Friedrich-Ebert-Stiftung Hessen.

Jakubowski, E., & Saltman, R.B. (2013). *The changing national role in health system governance: A case-based study of 11 European countries and Australia*. Observatory Studies Series 29. Copenhagen, Denmark: World Health Organization.

Kahlenberg, F.P., & Hoffmann, D. (2001). Sozialpolitik als Aufgabe zentraler Verwaltungen in Deutschland – ein verwaltungsgeschichtlicher Überblick 1945–1990. In Bundesministerium für Arbeit und Sozialordnung & Bundesarchiv (Eds.), *Geschichte der Sozialpolitik in Deutschland seit 1945* (vol. 1) (pp. 103–82). Baden-Baden, Germany: Nomos.

KBV. (2011). *Grunddaten zur Vertragsärztlichen Versorgung in Deutschland*. Berlin, Germany: Kassenärztliche Bundesvereinigung.

Lang, A. (2015). Germany. In K. Fierlbeck & H.A. Palley (Eds.), *Comparative health care federalism* (pp. 29–46). Farnham, UK: Ashgate.

Manow, P. (2004). *Federalism and the welfare state: The German case*. ZeS-Arbeitspapier 8/2004 [working paper]. Bremen, Zentrum für Sozialpolitik.

Manow, P. (2005). Germany: Co-operative federalism and the overgrazing of the fiscal commons. In H. Obinger, S. Leibfried, & F.G. Castles (Eds.), *Federalism and the welfare state: New World and European experiences* (pp. 222–62). Cambridge, UK: Cambridge University Press. https://doi.org/10.1017/CBO9780511491856.008

Neubauer, G. (2003). Zur Zukunft der dualen Finanzierung unter Wettbewerbsbedingungen. In M. Arnold, J. Klauber & H. Schellschmidt (Eds.), *Krankenhaus-Report 2002 – Krankenhaus im Wettbewerb* (pp. 71–92). Stuttgart, Germany: Schattauer.

Orlowski, U., & Wasem, J. (2003). *Gesundheitsreform 2004 – GKV-Modernisierungsgesetz (GMG)*. Heidelberg, Germany: Economica.

Pressel, H. (2012). *Der Gesundheitsfonds: Entstehung – Einführung – Weiterentwicklung – Folgen.* Wiesbaden, Germany: Springer VS.

Reiners, H. (1993). *Das Gesundheitsstrukturgesetz: Ein "Hauch von Sozialgeschichte"? Ein Werkstattbericht über eine gesundheitspolitische Weichenstellung.* WZB-Arbeitspapier 93–210 [working paper]. Berlin, Germany: Wissenschaftszentrum Berlin.

Requejo, F. (2010). Federalism and democracy: The case of minority nations. In M. Burgess & A. Gagnon (Eds.), *Federal democracies* (pp. 275–98). London, UK: Routledge.

Rosewitz, B., & Webber, D. (1990). *Reformversuche und Reformblockaden im deutschen Gesundheitswesen.* Frankfurt, Germany: Campus.

Statistisches Bundesamt. (2013). *Grunddaten der krankenhäuser 2011: Fachserie 12 Reihe 6.1.1.* Wiesbaden, Germany: Statistisches Bundesamt.

Stolleis, M. (2001). Sozialpolitik in Deutschland bis 1945. In Bundesministerium für Arbeit und Sozialordnung and Bundesarchiv (Ed.), Geschichte der *Sozialpolitik* in Deutschland seit 1945, vol. 1, 199–332. Baden-Baden, Germany: Nomos.

Welti, F. (2012). Die gesetzliche Krankenversicherung im Kräftefeld der Gesundheitspolitik. *Soziales Recht, 2*(3), 124–33.

Chapter Five

Pakistan: Extreme Decentralization

SANIA NISHTAR AND SANIYYA GAUHAR

Structural Features of the Federation

Introduction

The Islamic Republic of Pakistan is a federal republic consisting of four provinces – Punjab, Sindh, Khyber Pakhtunkhwa (KPK), and Balochistan – the federally administered tribal areas (FATA), and autonomous territories (Figure 5.1). The capital of Pakistan is Islamabad, which is a federal territory carved out of the Punjab. Pakistan is the sixth most populous country in the world, with an estimated population of 180.71 million (Ministry of Finance, 2012), and is culturally and ethnically diverse.

The 1973 Constitution of the Islamic Republic of Pakistan provides for a *federal parliamentary system* in which the provinces enjoy considerable autonomy, particularly after the passage of the 18th Constitutional Amendment on 20 April 2010, which devolved a large number of portfolios (including health) to the legislative and executive control of the provinces.

BRIEF POLITICAL HISTORY

In its seventy years of existence, Pakistan's political history and constitutional experience have been turbulent and dramatic. Pakistan came into being on 14 August 1947, in response to the demands of Muslims for an independent homeland, by the partition from British-ruled India of two Muslim-majority areas. After an initial period of eleven years of parliamentary democracy (during which time Pakistan was able to frame its first constitution in 1956 – nine years after independence), a military coup in 1958 led to martial law and the abrogation of the 1956 Constitution, ushering in a period of military rule for the next thirteen years under Field Marshal Ayub Khan. During this time, a

Figure 5.1 Map of Pakistan

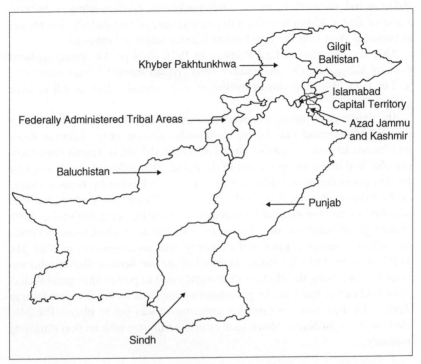

Khyber Pakhtunkhwa ⟶

Gilgit
Baltistan

Islamabad
Capital Territory

Azad Jammu
and Kashmir

Federally Administered Tribal Areas ⟶

Baluchistan ⟶

Punjab

Sindh

A version of this map first appeared in *The Lancet*, 2013; 381: 2194.

highly centralized, presidential form of government was introduced in 1962 under Pakistan's second constitution and after indirect presidential elections held in 1965. In 1969, Khan handed over control of the country to General Yahya Khan, commander-in-chief of the Pakistan Army, who instituted martial law with immediate effect and dissolved the National Assembly and the two provincial assemblies.[1]

In an attempt to effect a transition from military to civilian rule, Pakistan held its first general elections in 1970 (albeit under martial law) on the basis of "one man, one vote," which produced an overwhelming victory for the Awami League in East Pakistan headed by Sheikh Mujibur Rahman. This result was

---

1 Pakistan at that time had two provinces – East and West Pakistan; therefore, there were two provincial assemblies.

unpalatable to the ruling elite of West Pakistan and led to civil unrest in East Pakistan and ultimately to armed conflict in late 1971, culminating in the transition of East Pakistan into the independent state of Bangladesh. The former province of West Pakistan now became known simply as "Pakistan."

After the cessation of East Pakistan in 1971, Zulfiqar Ali Bhutto replaced General Yahya Khan as the country's first civilian martial law administrator, and in 1973, Pakistan's third constitution was enacted, which is still in force today.

The Bhutto government was overthrown in 1977 after a military coup led by General Mohammad Zia-ul-Haq, commander-in-chief of the Pakistan Army and the country was once again placed under martial law. In August 1988, General Zia died in a plane crash and in the decade that followed (1988–99), four civilian governments would come to power (two headed by Benazir Bhutto of the Pakistan Peoples Party [PPP] and two by Nawaz Sharif of the Pakistan Muslim League), but none of these completed their full term. In October 1999, Sharif's government was overthrown and the then army chief, General Pervez Musharraf, assumed control of the country until his resignation in 2008. The PPP headed by Asif Ali Zardari (husband of the late Benazir Bhutto, who was assassinated during the election campaign) came to power after general elections held earlier that year. Its government completed its full five-year term in April 2013, after which a caretaker government was put in place.[2] The 2013 elections brought Nawaz Sharif back as prime minister with an overwhelming majority.

The Federation

THE FEDERAL STRUCTURE

The 1973 Constitution is the supreme law of Pakistan and establishes a federal parliamentary system loosely based on the Westminster style. There are three pillars of the state – the legislature, the executive, and the judiciary – with institutions at both the national and the provincial level. The president is the head of state, and the prime minister is the head of government and chief executive of the federation.

Pakistan's federal legislature is its Parliament (Majlis-e-Shoora), which under the Constitution consists of both the president and a bicameral national legislature comprising the National Assembly (Lower House) and the Senate

---

2 The first author of this chapter, Sania Nishtar, served as a cabinet minister during this period.

(Upper House). After the 18th Amendment was passed in 2010, the president became more of a ceremonial figurehead representing the unity of the republic and must act on the advice of the prime minister or the cabinet, such advice being binding. The president is indirectly elected for a term of five years by a secret ballot through an electoral college comprising members of the Senate, the National Assembly, and the provincial assemblies. The National Assembly has a total of 342 seats, of which 272 are secured by means of direct elections based on universal adult suffrage, with provincial representation (seats) on the basis of population. Members of the National Assembly (MNAs) are elected for five-year terms. The provinces have an equal number of seats in the Senate, which has 104 indirectly elected members, of which 14 are elected from each of the provincial assemblies. Each senator has a term of six years, and elections for the Senate are held every three years for one-half of its members. Unlike the National Assembly, the Senate is not subject to dissolution.

The federal executive is headed by the prime minister, who is both the head of government and chief executive of the federation. The prime minister is elected by a simple majority vote of the National Assembly and is usually the head of the majority party or leader of a coalition government. The cabinet is appointed by the president on the advice of the prime minister and is collectively responsible to the Senate and National Assembly.

After the 18th Amendment's implementation in 2011, the federal Ministry of Health was abolished as the health portfolio devolved to the provinces. There was therefore no federal health minister until both the position and the ministry were restored in 2013 by the caretaker government.

THE PROVINCIAL STRUCTURE

The federal structure is largely replicated at the provincial level. Each of Pakistan's four provinces has its own provincial legislature known as a Provincial Assembly, but unlike the central legislature, the Provincial Assembly is unicameral. Its members are directly elected through universal adult franchise for a period of five years. The president (on the advice of the prime minister) appoints a governor for each province whose role largely mirrors that of the president.

The executive authority of the province is exercised in the name of the governor by the provincial government, consisting of the chief minister and the cabinet of provincial ministers (who act through the chief minister). The chief minister is elected by a simple majority vote of the Provincial Assembly. Ministers in the provincial cabinet are appointed by the governor from among members of the Provincial Assembly on the advice of the chief minister, whose advice is binding. The provincial cabinet is collectively responsible to the Provincial Assembly.

Each provincial government contains a health department or directorate with its own particular organizational arrangement. There is a provincial minister for health (unless the chief minister decides to retain the health portfolio), underneath whom is the secretary of health, the head bureaucrat.

LOCAL GOVERNMENT

Pakistan has had a somewhat chequered experience with local government and has, to date, been unable to establish a consistent, institutionalized system. Local government systems have tended to change when the government changes and have historically oscillated between highly centralized arrangements controlled by the provincial bureaucracy and some form of elected local bodies.[3] Part of the reason is that the Constitution does not explicitly set out any specific structure for local government (as it does in the cases of the federal and provincial governments), which seems to have provided successive governments with considerable flexibility in dissolving their predecessor's system and introducing a new system or arrangement that suits them. This, together with a lack of publicly available information, has created confusion and uncertainty as to the manner and method in which local government functions are being carried out. At present, there is no homogenized setup, and although recently enacted legislation provides for various local councils to carry out some health functions, this is currently being undertaken at the provincial and federal levels.

The Council of Common Interests

The Constitution also provides for the establishment of a Council of Common Interests (CCI), which is an *executive* body headed by the prime minister and consisting of the four provincial chief ministers and three members of the federal government nominated by the prime minister. Its purpose is to foster a harmonious working relationship between the federal government and the provinces. More importantly, the CCI is empowered to formulate and regulate policies related to matters set out in Part II of the Federal Legislative List (FLL) in the Constitution. In theory, the CCI is an important body for the provinces to air their grievances against the federation or each other and for seeking a solution to these grievances.

---

3 In general, civilian governments have been reluctant to devolve power to local bodies, whereas military regimes have favoured structured and more decentralized arrangements (see Bossert & Mitchell, 2010).

Distribution of Power between the Federation and the Provinces

Since its enactment in 1973, one of the hallmarks of the Constitution was that it essentially recognized the principle of decentralization and provided the basis for a distribution of power between the federal and provincial governments. The distribution of legislative power between Parliament and the provincial assemblies is set out in the Constitution in the Federal Legislative List (in Schedule 4). The FLL is divided into two parts. Parliament has exclusive power to legislate on all matters contained in Part I of the FLL, such as defence, public debt, external affairs, and currency. Part II of the FLL allows for some provincial participation as the CCI is empowered to formulate and regulate policies on all matters set out therein and also to exercise supervision and control over related institutions. Matters such as railways, electricity, minerals, oil, natural gas, regulation and the census are listed here.

Any matter *not* listed in the FLL falls within the exclusive legislative purview of the provinces. Since health and matters related to health are *not* listed in the FLL, health legislative authority was constitutionally defined as predominantly a provincial subject. However, health information is a Part I FLL subject, whereas regulation is a Part II FLL subject. This was the basis of the mandate of the federal/national-level health ministry established by the 2013 caretaker government, as described later in this chapter.

Under the 1973 Constitution, in addition to the FLL, there was also defined a Concurrent Legislative List (CLL). The CLL listed forty-seven subjects (including health) that could be legislated upon by both the federal government and the provincial governments. In the case of any ambiguity or contradictions, federal law was to prevail. The CLL was used by the federation to assert its policies in health until it was abolished by the 18th Amendment.

The rationale for the centre having concurrent control was that exclusive legislative authority by the provinces was felt to be undesirable, as they did not have the institutional capacity to exclusively deal with these matters; in the event of a situation arising whereby the centre would have to deal with these on a national level, it retained the power to do so.

Recent Constitutional Developments – the 18th Amendment

In the years prior to the passage of the 18th Constitutional Amendment, political discourse had centred on curtailing the powers of the president, which had increased over the years, particularly under the two previous military governments, when the country had moved towards a more centralized, presidential system. There had also been considerable clamour for greater provincial autonomy. The preamble of the 18th Amendment states it purpose: "The people of Pakistan have relentlessly struggled for democracy and for attaining the ideals of a Federal, Islamic, democratic, parliamentary and modern progressive welfare State, wherein the rights of the citizens are secured and the Provinces have equitable share in the Federation." The second stated purpose was to nullify the 17th Constitutional Amendment and the Legal Framework Order 2002 passed by the previous military government of General Pervez Musharraf.

The 18th Amendment, passed unanimously by Parliament on 20 April 2010, effected a sweeping reorganization in the distribution of power at both the national and provincial levels (Government of Pakistan, 2011). Containing a total of 102 amendments, this piece of legislation significantly altered power sharing between the federal and provincial governments in Pakistan's federal system. The aim of the lawmakers was to strengthen parliamentary democracy, which they felt had been eroded over the years by changes previous military governments had made to the Constitution; such changes had resulted in a more centralized system, which severely hampered the smooth progress of democratic government. The 18th Amendment sought to redress this situation by reducing the powers of the president and strengthening the executive power of the prime minister (a power that had been repeatedly usurped and curtailed throughout Pakistan's history), and devolving a large number of portfolios to the exclusive legislative and executive control of the provinces, thereby granting provincial autonomy over these subjects.

The 18th Amendment abolished the CLL in its entirety. As a result, seventeen federal ministries – including the Ministry of Health (MoH) – were perceived to be redundant and were hence abolished (Nishtar & Mehboob, 2011). Their functions were either given to the provinces or were scattered across other ministries at the federal level. Further details are discussed later in this chapter.

However, three years after the 18th Amendment, the MoH was re-established by the caretaker government in 2013 as it was recognized that some form of central coordination was needed lest health policy became too nebulous and health functions unsynchronized.[4]

The Decentralization of Health

The Health System: A Snapshot

Pakistan has a mixed health system where public provision of services coexists alongside a predominant private market in health care (Nishtar, 2010a, 2010b).

---

4 One of the authors (Sania Nishtar) was the caretaker federal minister responsible for re-establishing the Ministry of Health.

The public-sector health care delivery system comprises 965 public hospitals, 12,000 first-level care facilities (FLCFs), and 90,000 community-based female Lady Health Workers; the last group provides family planning and reproductive health services door-to-door in Pakistan's rural areas, covering more than 50 per cent of the population (Oxford Policy Management, 2011). Low salaries in the public system manifest in the form of a number of individual coping strategies, such as absenteeism and moonlighting in the private sector. These are exacerbated by absence of regulatory controls and quality assurance mechanisms, poor management, and limited accountability in governance.

According to population-based health service access data, three-quarters of the services are delivered in the private sector (Federal Bureau of Statistics, 2012). However, the private system is undocumented and unregulated and comprises a plethora of actors. It is heterogeneous in terms of the service facilities, the qualification of providers, and the system of medicine followed.

In terms of health financing, the public sector is responsible for 0.9 per cent of the country's GDP, and 78.08 per cent of the population pays out-of-pocket at the point of service. Complex governance challenges and under-investment in health have hampered progress. Significant policy distortions are evident, as in the case of human resource discrepancies: for example, physicians outnumber nurses and midwives by a factor of 2 to 1. The high number of spurious medicines is indicative of deep-seated regulatory problems. Recent analysis of the health system shows that more than seventy years after its inception, Pakistan's health system has been unable to achieve the three health system goals – adequate and equitable health status, fairness in financing, and responsiveness (Nishtar, Bhutta, et al., 2013; Nishtar, Boerma, et al., 2013).

In relation to outcomes, Pakistan has shown some health status improvements over the last sixty-five years, but key health indicators lag behind twelve other peer countries. The country has the third highest rates of maternal, fetal, and child mortality globally and has made slow progress in achieving Millennium Development Goals (MDG) 4 and 5 targets (Bhutta et al., 2013). Non-communicable diseases (NCDs) have become the major cause of morbidity and mortality, leading to an annual loss of over US$3.5 billion in productive life years (Jafar et al., 2013).

Health Decentralization in Pakistan

Historically, many attempts have been made to decentralize the health care system in Pakistan. Examples include the 1990s financial management decentralization of health at the *tehsil* level, a level between province and district (Collins,

Omar, & Tarin, 2002); the Sheikhupura Project (UNICEF, 1994); the 1996–7 establishment of District Health Authorities and District Health Management Teams; the 1998 District Health Government reform initiatives (Collins, Omar, & Tarin, 2002); and the local government initiative of 2001 (Cheema, Khwaja, & Qadir, 2006). As noted, the 18th Amendment, on the other hand, was in effect a reform of Pakistan's federal system, which altered power sharing in the federal provincial polity.

The 18th Amendment to the Constitution devolved seventeen "subjects," including health, to the provinces in Pakistan's federal system. In the wake of this decision, it was perceived that the federal government had only a limited role in these areas, and therefore, their corresponding ministries, including the MoH, were abolished. Other health-relevant changes brought about by the 18th Amendment are summarized in Table 5.1.

After the MoH's abolition, several institutions of health, particularly those related to service delivery, were devolved to the provinces, but many remained at the federal level as per constitutional provisions outlined in the Federal Legislative Lists. However, these were scattered across nine different ministries and divisions, to which they reported (Figure 5.2). Fragmentation of health care posed many problems, including lack of coordination both at the federal level and at the intergovernmental level, interagency turf tensions, undermining of federal-level decision-making ability because of the information-evidence-policy disconnect, and lack of clarity about responsibilities, with resulting difficulty for international partners (Nishtar, 2011). It should be noted that because of the unique history of Pakistan and the extreme constitutionally driven process of decentralization, we include here a decision space map for the national government and note that some functions are defined by constitution or by negotiation, limiting both central and subnational governments.

Lack of clarity in drug regulatory arrangements and rivalry between the provinces over control of the drug regulatory turf led to an impasse for over a year, during which there was effectively no drug regulatory arrangements in place. Part of the confusion arose because the mandate to create regulatory authorities in general was given to the federal government by the 18th Amendment, but in cases where the subject to be regulated was devolved – "drugs and medicine" in this case – both the federal government and the provinces claimed to have the mandate. In this particular case, the confusion continued for over a year during consultations. It was only after more than a hundred people died in the Isotab drug scandal (Nishtar, 2012) that the provinces conceded regulatory authority in favour of the federal government by virtue of a constitutional instrument, Article 144, through which provinces can ask the federal government to perform a function on their behalf.

Table 5.1 Pakistan's 18th Constitutional Amendment: Health-relevant changes

Area of change in the constitution	Nature of the change	Implication for the health sector
Concurrent Legislative List		
Abolition of the Concurrent Legislative List	The following entries were deleted: "Drugs and medicines"; "Poisons and dangerous drugs"; "Prevention of the extension from one province to another, of infectious or contagious diseases …"; "Mental illness and mental retardation …"; "Environmental pollution and ecology", "Population planning"; "Welfare of labor, conditions of labor …"; "Legal, medical and other professions", "Inquiries and statistics"	It was inferred that with deletion of these entries, the federal government has no role in the health sector. However, an independent report outlined that the Constitution still provided space for retaining national roles federally, with the exception of "Drugs and medicines."
Federal Legislative List		
Shifting of an entry from the CLL to the Federal Legislative List (FLL), Part II	"Legal, medical and other professions" was shifted from the CLL to Part II of the FLL	Health workforce regulation is now dealt with federally, albeit with formulation of policies by the CCI
Insertion of a new entry into the FLL, Part I	"International treaties, conventions and agreements and international arbitration"	International agreements are totally in the federal/ national purview
Shifting of an entry from Part I to Part II of the FLL	"National planning and economic coordination, including planning and coordination of scientific and technological research"	Through this, the provinces have been empowered to play a role in an area/subject which was previously not their mandate
Amendments in Article 144	This enables any one provincial assembly by resolution to empower the Parliament to enact legislation to regulate matters not contained in the FLL	This represents one constitutional mechanism for overcoming issues arising as a consequence of the massive devolution authority to the provinces through omission of the CLL and was brought in effect when mandating drug regulation
Amendments in Article 270	Article 270AA(6) saves all laws and other legal instruments having the force of law with respect to any matter contained in the omitted CLL, which were enacted prior to the 18th Amendment. These laws continue to remain in force until altered, repealed, or amended by what is referred to as the "competent authority."	Existing health-related laws will continue to be in force. However, while the 18th Amendment "saved" laws, it may have transferred the power to alter, repeal, or amend laws in favour of the provinces, which may now be "competent authority" as referred to in Article 270AA(6).
Abolition of the Ministry of Health	The Ministry of Health was abolished and there was no central/federal institutional structure for health in the country	Fragmentation of national health functions across seven other provincial domains

Figure 5.2 Health fragmentation in the aftermath of abolition of Pakistan's Ministry of Health

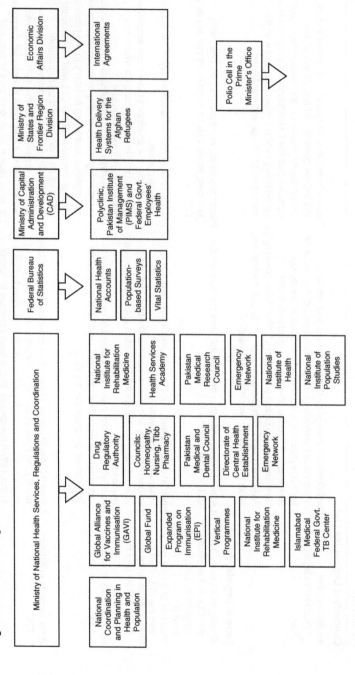

Leading up to March 2013, matters significantly worsened after a donor consortium blocked a tranche of support for supporting measles Supplementary Immunization Days, citing lack of clarity in institutional coordination arrangements. Donors as well as provinces had been calling for a central coordinating arrangement for health at the federal level. A multi-partner donor mission also concluded its reports with the same recommendations in 2013 (WHO, World Bank, DFID, & USAID-TAUH, 2012). During the interim government in 2013, the Ministry of Health was re-established. (Nishtar, 2013).

The constitutional rationale of the new Ministry of Health, its mandate, remit, and functions, which stem from the Legislative Lists, have been stipulated (Nishtar, 2013) and are outlined later in this chapter.

Assessing Health System Decentralization and Centralization

In this section, the current degree of decentralization within Pakistan's health system will be examined using the decision space analysis discussed earlier in this book (Bossert, 1998). Tables 5.2 and 5.3 outline the degree of decision space in Pakistan at the federal and provincial levels after the 18th Amendment to the Constitution.

The decision space approach allows us to disaggregate the functions over which officials have a defined range of discretion, rather than seeing decentralization as a single transfer or a block of authority and responsibility (Bossert, 1998). The decision space map was used to analyse the relationship between three dimensions of decentralization – decentralized authority (referred to as "decision space"), institutional capacities, and accountability to local officials – among district-level, health sector decision makers after the local government reform of 2001. The results show that decision makers were using decision space to differing degrees despite being under a single decentralization regime and adhering to similar rules across provinces.

Because of the current nature of administrative arrangements at the local government level, decision space was not gauged at that level for this analysis. Rather than an analysis of decision-making at the local level for which this tool has traditionally been employed, this analysis will focus on federal versus provincial decision space after the 18th Constitutional Amendment.

Gauging Decision Space in the Pakistan Health System

As noted before, the federal-level decision space is defined by two Legislative Lists in Pakistan's Constitution that enumerate "subjects." Part I of the FLL outlines mandates in a purely federal purview, for which the competent authority is now the

Table 5.2 Decision space for federal government in Pakistan's health system after enactment of the 18th Constitutional Amendment

Function	Indicator	Range of Choice		
		Narrow	Moderate	Wide
Financing				
Sources of revenue	Federal transfers to the provinces under the National Finance Commission Award	One-line fiscal transfers are made to the provinces under an agreed formula of fiscal sharing		
Expenditure allocation for subjects that are federal	Federal Public Sector Development Program allocations to federal institutions			Federal government can internally decide how it wants to earmark resources in the federal envelope for health
Expenditure allocation for subjects that are provincial	Provincial Public Sector Development Program allocations	This is solely a provincial subject		
Insurance	Constitutionally defined federal mandate in insurance prerogative		Constitution empowers the federal government to launch insurance schemes for residents in the federal territory and the specially administered areas. The federal government can also launch an insurance scheme in a province if the province fails to launch it in the interest of protecting its citizens.	

Social protection	Constitutionally defined federal mandate to risk-protect people from impoverishment	Federal government has its own social protection agency. However, social protection is a provincial subject.
Service organization and delivery		
Required programs	Rules on what services must be delivered	Federal government has limited role in outlining required program to the provinces, which are autonomous in this area. However, if there is an international agreement to be complied with, then the federal government has a role. Until 2015 federal government made it conditional for provinces to run certain preventive programs and underwrote their cost.
Payment mechanisms	Rules on payments to hospitals and physicians	Already defined but flexibility exists to modify these
Hospital autonomy	Choice of how hospitals are governed, organized, and paid	Federal hospitals exist under different arrangements, but the flexibility exists to modify arrangements
Norms and standard-setting for quality	Constitutionally defined prerogative	This is a shared mandate between the provinces and the federal government

(Continued)

Table 5.2 Decision space for federal government in Pakistan's health system after enactment of the 18th Constitutional Amendment (Continued)

Function	Indicator	Range of Choice		
		Narrow	Moderate	Wide
Human resources				
Salaries	Choice of salary range	Already defined according to civil service rules		
Contracting	Contracting non-permanent staff			Federal government can take contract appointees
Civil service	Hiring and firing	Under civil service rules this is tightly regulated		
Governance rules				
Policymaking mandate	Extent to which the federal government is empowered to formulate policy	Federal government has a narrow mandate in health		
Regulatory mandate for drugs and medicines	Constitutionally defined regulatory prerogative			Drug regulation is a federal subject as returned from the provinces by agreement
Regulatory mandate relevant to human resource	Constitutionally defined regulatory prerogative	This mandate is shared with the provinces. Therefore it is a subject of the federation. The federal government has a narrow mandate in this area without provincial concurrence		

Regulatory mandate relevant to services and quality	Constitutionally defined regulatory prerogative	This is a provincial subject
Administration of government service delivery institutions	Government of Pakistan Rules of Business—defined administrative prerogative	Jurisdiction over government institutions that are either limited to the federal territory or are "national" and therefore could not be devolved to the provinces
Coordination	Government of Pakistan Rules of Business—defined mandate to coordinate	National planning and economic coordination between provinces for scientific and technological research and communicable diseases and epidemic control
International agreements and regulations	Constitutionally defined regulatory prerogative	Dealings and agreements with foreign countries and international organizations in the field of health. Adoption of International Health Regulations; Registration, accreditation, and regulations related to HR.

(Continued)

Table 5.2 Decision space for federal government in Pakistan's health system after enactment of the 18th Constitutional Amendment (Continued)

Function	Indicator	Range of Choice		
		Narrow	Moderate	Wide
Other				
Health information	Constitutionally defined federal mandate related to health information			Health information collection, consolidation, analysis. This includes management information systems, disease surveillance, epidemiological surveillance, registries, and other mechanisms of health information.
Research	Constitutionally defined federal mandate related to research			Oversight of bioethical practices in health research
Standard-setting in higher education and research	Government of Pakistan Rules of Business– defined mandate to set standards			Standards in institutions for higher education and research; graduate and postgraduate public health institutions

Table 5.3 Provincial-level decision space in Pakistan's health system after enactment of the 18th Constitutional Amendment

Function	Indicator	Range of Choice		
		Narrow	Moderate	Wide
Financing				
Sources of revenue	Resource mobilization	Provinces have the mandate to mobilize revenue, but owing to limited capacity have to rely on federal grants under the National Finance Commission Award		
Expenditure allocation for health	Expenditure on health as a % of the federal government's National Finance Commission Award to the provinces as well as indigenously mobilized revenue			Provinces have full control to allocate resources to different sectors
Insurance	Constitutionally defined mandate			Provincial responsibility and prerogative
Social protection	Constitutionally defined mandate to risk-protect people from impoverishment			Provincial responsibility and mandate

(Continued)

Table 5.3 Provincial-level decision space in Pakistan's health system after enactment of the 18th Constitutional Amendment (Continued)

Function	Indicator	Range of Choice		
		Narrow	Moderate	Wide
Service organization and delivery				
Required programs	Rules on what services must be delivered			Provincial governments can decide on the nature of essential services
Payment mechanisms	Rules on payments to hospitals and physicians		Already defined but flexibility exists to modify these	
Hospital autonomy	Choice of how hospitals are governed, organized, and paid			Provincial governments can decide on managing hospitals in any way they deem suitable, including grant of autonomy
Human resources				
Salaries	Choice of salary range	Already defined according to service rules		
Contracting	Contracting non-permanent staff			Provincial government can take contract appointees
Civil service	Hiring and firing	Under civil service rules, this is tightly regulated		
Governance rules				
Policymaking mandate	Extent to which the provincial government is empowered to formulate policy			Provinces have the prerogative to formulate health policies relevant to their context

Function	Federal mandate			
Regulatory mandate for drugs and medicines	Constitutionally defined regulatory prerogative	Provinces have given this mandate to the federal government		
Regulatory mandate relevant to human resources	Constitutionally defined regulatory prerogative		This mandate is shared with the federal government; therefore it is a subject of the federation	
Regulatory mandate relevant to services and quality	Constitutionally defined regulatory prerogative			Provinces have the mandate to regulate quality in subjects that have been devolved
Administration of government service delivery institutions	Government of Pakistan Rules of Business–defined administrative prerogative			Provinces have full control over their institutions
Coordination	Government of Pakistan Rules of Business–defined mandate to coordinate		Provinces have the mandate to coordinate the districts. The federal government is responsible for coordination between provinces and interprovincial convening through the institution of the Council of Common Interests.	
Standard-setting in higher education and research	Government of Pakistan Rules of Business–defined mandate to set standards	This is a federal subject		

(Continued)

Table 5.3 Provincial-level decision space in Pakistan's health system after enactment of the 18th Constitutional Amendment (Continued)

Function	Indicator	Range of Choice		
		Narrow	Moderate	Wide
Governance rules				
Standard-setting in quality	Constitutionally defined prerogative		This is a shared mandate between the provinces and the federal government	
International agreements and regulations	Constitutionally defined regulatory prerogative	This is a federal subject		
Other				
Health information	Constitutionally defined mandate related to health information	Only related to collection and passing on to the central hub		
Research	Constitutionally defined mandate related to research	Federal mandate		

Ministry of National Health Services, Regulation, and Coordination. For subjects enumerated in Part II of the FLL, the CCI is the competent authority. These are subjects of the federation (as defined by the CCI) and not the federal government.

POLICYMAKING

The space for federal-level policymaking in health stems from the Legislative Lists. In health-systems-related functions that have a truly national character – health information, regulation, disease security, compliance with international agreements, interprovincial coordination, and trade in health – the mandate to formulate policy is clearly with the federal government. While these functions are important, it is obvious that there is a lack of mechanisms to develop national policy through assertion of national objectives and norms and standards for the entire nation, as well as mechanisms for coordination among subnational units, except perhaps through the CCI.

One of the specific roles of the central government in other federal systems is ensuring equity among the subnational units. This can be achieved by supporting the weaker units with financial and/or normative support and creating incentives that can act as a catalyst for performance enhancement. In Pakistan there are two bottlenecks in this respect: the absence of a monitoring mechanism, and the lack of a fiscal instrument that can tie performance to incentives. The federal government through its judicial authority could also intervene to preserve national equity and solidarity in case there is litigation between providers and users from different provinces; however, these mechanisms are currently lacking in Pakistan.

REGULATION

Regulation in the health sector can be relevant to quality, price, or numbers in the domain of health services delivery, medical education, human resources, and medicines and technologies. In most federated countries, regulation is a national/federal subject as it obviates the need for agreements regarding acceptance of each other's standards. Constitutional covenants stipulating subnational trade usually serve as the basis for a federal mandate in the area. The case of the United States of America is illustrative, where the commerce clause has served as the basis for much national-level health regulation, including drug regulation.

Regulation is a federal subject in Pakistan, with the mandate emanating from Entry 6 of the FLL, Part II, and interprovincial trade of services is guaranteed by Article 155 of the Constitution. This gives the federal government the powers to establish federal-level regulatory authorities, albeit with concurrence at the CCI. Several regulatory authorities are therefore in the federal jurisdiction.

In keeping with this constitutional mandate, several health regulatory authorities are attached to the re-established federal Ministry of Health. The Drug Regulatory Authority (DRA) is the most important in this regard. Federal-level decision space should be used effectively to overcome some of the critical distortions which currently plague drug regulatory arrangements, as the present arrangements do not command confidence by any measure and need to be radically altered for true, robust, and independent regulatory oversight. In addition, the Drug and Medicines Policy 1998 and the Drug Act 1976 need to be updated.

HEALTH FINANCING

Formula-based resource transfers occur from the national divisible pool of revenue at several levels; the formula takes into account population, inverse population density, and poverty. At the highest level, the National Finance Commission (NFC) Award divides the available revenue pool between the four provinces and the federal government according to a predetermined formula, which was revised in 2009 and takes into account population and the level of provincial development to ensure equitable per capita spending among provinces. Provincial Finance Commission Awards distribute resources from the provincial to the local government level. The modalities of this system have not changed with the 18th Amendment, except for the size of provincial allocations, which has increased significantly in the seventh NFC. The provinces are free to earmark funding to sectors and areas according to their own priorities. Provinces have capacity constraints with respect to revenue mobilization and rely on the federal government for tax collection. Even in the case of the services tax, which is a provincial mandate, provinces rely on the federal government for collection on their behalf. Within the first five years of the 18th Amendment, until 2015, provinces got earmarked additional resources for vertical public health programs, until such time that their own capacity was developed to mobilize needed revenue. This allocation amounted to less than 5 per cent of the total provincial health budget.

The decisions about health financing arrangements, pooling mechanisms, and purchasing are now provincial prerogatives. This makes sense, as these are not independent of service delivery decisions and have to be made in view of existing arrangements or the manner in which service delivery is envisaged to evolve as a result of concomitant reform.

However there are three areas where the federal government has decision space. The first of these was of a temporary nature, as the federal government agreed to finance the vertical public health programs until 2015; after that, the provinces were expected fund the vertical programs themselves.

The second is relevant to the broader question of earmarking of revenues for health. As of 2017, taxation is a federal function since provinces have given the federal government their mandate to mobilize resources. Therefore, innovative financing options will continue to be a federal decision-making prerogative until provinces develop their own capacity to mobilize revenue. It must be noted that revenue allocation under the NFC Award is a federal responsibility. The 18th Amendment has not changed that.

Third, Entry 29 in Part I of the FLL is the only entry on financing directly related to a specific aspect of health financing. This can be the basis for introducing a federally led health insurance or a social insurance scheme, if needed and not initiated at the provincial level. All other health-financing-related functions stand devolved to the provinces.

SERVICE DELIVERY

The space for decision-making in relation to service delivery is now fully in the provincial domain unless there are service delivery institutions that relate to the federal capital territory. The federal government had, prior to the abolition of the Ministry of Health and for several years running, invested in a range of service delivery institutions, under a specific entry, which enabled it to create large hospitals on provincial territory: "Federal agencies and institutes for the following purposes, that is to say, for research, for professional or technical training, or for the promotion of special studies" (FLL, Part 1, Entry 16). These hospitals have now been devolved to the provinces since service delivery is a "devolved subject," but since their transitional arrangements were not carefully managed, they continue to be plagued by problems, especially in relation to human resources matters – retirement benefits, promotions, and career structures.

INFORMATION COMMUNICATION TECHNOLOGY IN HEALTH

Information communication technology (ICT) is a federal mandate, to the extent of formulation of policy; however, since it is deeply linked with relevant sectors, provincial implementation and mainstreaming is expected. Pakistan has many health-relevant ICT strengths – over 119 million mobile users, a national repository of identities, a national poverty registry, the central repository of health providers, a burgeoning mobile money sector, and a database of registered providers. These capabilities can be leveraged for innovative entry points to universal coverage reform. The use of technology can bring significant value to many health system domains by improving efficiency, controlling costs, reducing human errors, facilitating new services, and improving connectivity. It can also assist with minimizing leakages and pilferages from the health system. Appropriate use of technology can help revolutionize learning, continuing medical education (CME), and information dissemination. The space to mainstream changes in this area is in the federal as well as the provincial purview; however, ICT per se is a federal mandate.

HUMAN RESOURCES IN HEALTH

The 18th Amendment does not alter federal functions related to human resources insofar as regulatory and standard-setting roles are concerned. However, the exercise of federal executive authority in this respect will now be subject to provincial concurrence and policy oversight at the forum of CCI. Related institutions such as regulatory authorities (e.g., Pakistan Medical and Dental Council, Pakistan Nursing Council) are also subject to supervision and control by CCI. The post–18th Amendment problematic area in human resources relates to the status of people who were employees of institutions that have been devolved to the provinces. Major hospitals, under federal jurisdiction prior to the 18th Amendment, were transferred to the provinces, but their employees continue to be federal employees now on "deputation" to the provinces and paid from the federal treasury. As a result, confusion looms around promotions and retirement benefits, with resulting difficulties for former federal government employees. These contentious matters require careful management by both orders of government.

INTERNATIONAL AGREEMENTS

Pakistan is a signatory to a number of international agreements in the health sector. Most of these are not legally binding, but some have obligatory reporting requirements, as in the case of the Millennium Development Goals. The Constitution by virtue of Entry 2 of Part I of the FLL gives the federal government the mandate to enter into and subsequently deal with international agreements. However, since the 18th Amendment, the actual implementation of these agreements is now in the provincial domain.

Conclusion

There can be many levers of health systems reform; in the case of Pakistan, decentralization has been an "inadvertent" entry point. With the 18th Amendment, reform has been forced on the health sector in Pakistan, and the basic shift towards more provincial authority and responsibility in the health sector is likely to be retained. But the reform went too far in decentralizing functions; in fact, it led to an abdication of responsibility on the part of the federal government and stripped the federal government and the federation of the needed institutions and instruments to play its constitutionally granted role. Also, without local government reform, it also led to centralization of power in provinces and has, therefore, not helped with further decentralization to local government. Since 2013, some arrangements have been slowly getting back in shape. A Ministry of Health has been re-established with a mandate that conforms to the stipulations set in the Constitution. Although it was re-established by a caretaker government, the subsequent elected political government has assumed ownership of the change. The ministry is not likely to be rolled back. By and large, provinces do not view the federal ministry as threatening their mandate. However, there are a number of key imperatives for the steps ahead. In addition to strengthening the federal ministry, it is critical to invest in capacity building of provincial departments of health, who now have the bulk of responsibility related to health; this will entail a major effort. Also it is imperative to give more authority to local government arrangements, to effectively implement devolution in its true spirit.

REFERENCES

Bhutta, Z.A., Hafiz, A., Rizvi, A., Ali, N., Khan, A., Ahmad, F., . . . Jafarey, S.N. (2013). The enigma of reproductive, material, newborn and child health in Pakistan: Challenges and opportunities. *Lancet, 381*(9884), 2207–18. https://doi.org/10.1016/S0140-6736(12)61999-0

Bossert, T. (1998). Analyzing the decentralization of health systems in developing countries: Decision space, innovation and performance. *Social Science & Medicine, 47*(10), 1513–27. https://doi.org/10.1016/S0277-9536(98)00234-2

Bossert, T.J., & Mitchell, A.D. (2010). Health sector decentralization and local decision-making: Decision space, institutional capacities and accountability in Pakistan. *Social Science & Medicine, 72*(1), 39–48.

Cheema, A., Khwaja, A.I., & Qadir, A. (2006). Local government reforms in Pakistan: Context, content and causes. In P. Bardhan & D. Mookherjee (Eds.), *Decentralization and local governance in developing countries: A comparative perspective* (pp. 257–84). Cambridge, MA: MIT Press.

Collins, C.D., Omar, M., & Tarin, E. (2002). Decentralization, healthcare and policy process in the Punjab, Pakistan in the 1990s. *International Journal of Health Planning and Management, 17*(2), 123–46. https://doi.org/10.1002/hpm.657

Federal Bureau of Statistics. (2012). *Pakistan social and living standards measurements survey, 2010–11*. Islamabad, Pakistan: Government of Pakistan.

Government of Pakistan. (2011). 18th Constitutional Amendment, Constitution of the Islamic Republic of Pakistan. https://www.scribd.com/doc/30269950

/18th-Amendment-in-the-Constitution-of-Pakistan-Complete-Text. Retrieved 12 December 2011.

Jafar, T.H., Haaland, B.A., Rahman, A., Razzak, J., Bilger, M., Naghavi, M., … & Hyder, A. (2013). Non-communicable diseases and injuries in Pakistan: Strategic priorities. *Lancet, 381*(9885), 2281–90. https://doi.org/10.1016/S0140-6736(13)60646-7

Ministry of Finance. (2012). *Pakistan Economic Survey, 2011/12.* Islamabad, Pakistan: Government of Pakistan.

Nishtar, S. (2010a). *Choked pipes: Reforming Pakistan's mixed health system.* Oxford, UK: Oxford University Press.

Nishtar, S. (2010b). Mixed health systems syndrome. *Bulletin of the World Health Organization, 88*(1), 74–5. https://doi.org/10.2471/BLT.09.067868. http://www.who.int/bulletin/volumes/88/1/09-067868/en/

Nishtar, S. (2011). Health and the 18th Amendment: Retaining national functions in devolution. Heartfile. http://www.heartfile.org/pdf/HEALTH_18AM_FINAL.pdf. Retrieved 1 September 2016.

Nishtar, S. (2012, March). Pakistan's deadly cocktail of substandard drugs. *Lancet, 379*(9821), 1084–5. http://dx.doi.org/10.1016/S0140-6736(12)60277-3

Nishtar, S. (2013) Handover Papers: Towards improving governance. Government of Pakistan. http://www.sanianishtar.info/pdfs/HOP-Compendium_Final.pdf

Nishtar, S., Bhutta, Z.A., Jafar, T.H., Ghaffar, A., Akhtar, T., Bengali, K., Isa, Q.A., & Rahim, E. (2013). Health reform in Pakistan: A call to action. *Lancet, 381*(9885), 2291–7. https://doi.org/10.1016/S0140-6736(13)60813-2

Nishtar, S., Boerma, T., Amjad, S., Alam, A.Y., Khalid, F., ul Haq, I., & Mirza, Y.A. (2013). Pakistan's health system: Performance and prospects after the 18th Constitutional Amendment. *Lancet, 381*(9884), 2193–206. https://doi.org/10.1016/S0140-6736(13)60019-7

Nishtar, S., & Mehboob, A.B. (2011). Pakistan prepares to abolish Ministry of Health. *Lancet, 378*(9792), 648–9. https://doi.org/10.1016/S0140-6736(11)60606-5

Oxford Policy Management. (2011). Lady Health Worker Programme external evaluation of the National Programme for Family Planning and Primary Health Care. Summary of Results.

UNICEF. (1994). *The state of public sector primary health care services, district Sheikhupura, Punjab, Pakistan. Bamako Initiative Technical Report Series.* New York, NY: UNICEF.

WHO, World Bank, DFID, & USAID-TAUH. (2012). Devolution of the heath sector following the 18th Amendment to the Constitution of Pakistan: Opportunities and challenges. Islamabad, Pakistan: World Health Organization.

Chapter Six

Federalism, Interdependence, and the Health Care System in South Africa

LAETITIA C. RISPEL AND JULIA MOORMAN

Structural Features of South Africa

In July 2017, the Republic of South Africa (RSA), located at the southern end of the African continent, had a population of 56.5 million (Statistics South Africa, 2017). The country is divided into nine provinces, as shown in Figure 6.1.

The South African rights-based Constitution was promulgated in December 1996, two years after the country's first democratic elections in 1994 (Republic of South Africa, 1996). This document drastically changed the organization and administrative divisions of the country. A long history of colonization and apartheid had deeply fragmented the country and created originally a number of "homelands" (Ciskei, Transkei, Bophuthatswana, Venda, Gazankulu, KaNgwane, KwaNdebele, KwaZulu, Lebowa, and QwaQwa) and four provinces (Cape of Good Hope, Transvaal, Orange Free State, and Natal). The "homelands" were territories set aside, within the borders of South Africa, for black African inhabitants along ethnic lines. In theory these homelands were expected to be "independent and self-governing." In reality, a lack of economic infrastructure, resources, and legitimacy and entrenched racism and discrimination ensured their dependence on the national government. There were also numerous municipalities – transitional metropolitan councils, local councils, and transitional rural councils, all fragmented by race (Buhlungu & Atkinson, 2007).

The 1996 Constitution created one democratic state and three spheres of government – national, provincial, and local government. The three levels of government are all constitutionally recognized and are envisaged as "distinctive, interdependent and interrelated" (Republic of South Africa, 1996). Nine provinces were created – Eastern Cape, Free State, Gauteng, KwaZulu Natal, Limpopo, Mpumalanga, Northern Cape, North West, and Western Cape

Figure 6.1 Map of South Africa and its provinces

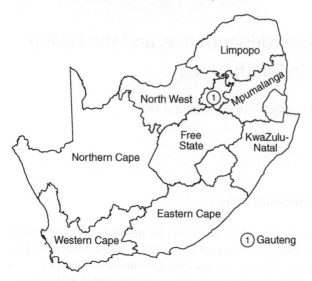

(Republic of South Africa, 1996). The local sphere of government consists of a multitude of municipalities[1] with the constitutional right to govern within their geographical boundaries. Neither national nor provincial government may compromise a municipality's right to exercise its powers. The structure of local government is further refined through specific legislation. The 1998 Local Government Demarcation Act and the 1998 Local Government Municipal Structures Act make provision for the establishment of various types of municipalities and their functions and powers (Cameron, 2006). Municipalities were defined in three categories – metropolitan (cities or category A municipalities), district (more than one town or category C municipalities), and local (small towns or category B municipalities) (Cameron, 2006).

The functions of the three spheres of government are outlined clearly in the Constitution. The National Parliament consists of two houses of parliament,

---

1 Municipalities are geographical areas under the control of local government. Although the boundaries of a health district are coterminous with (i.e., the same as) municipal boundaries, the functions of a municipality are determined by the Constitution, whereas the health district is an administrative demarcation by the Department of Health.

the National Assembly and the National Council of Provinces (NCOP), and is responsible for passing national legislation affecting the entire country (Republic of South Africa, 1996). The constitutional mandate of the NCOP is to ensure that provincial interests are taken into account in the national sphere of government, both through participation in the national legislative process and by providing a national forum for consideration of issues affecting provinces (https://www.parliament.gov.za/, accessed 13 August 2016). The goal is to achieve synergy between the two spheres of government on matters of concurrent competence (Republic of South Africa, 1996). The NCOP consists of ninety provincial delegates, or ten delegates for each of the nine provinces. A provincial delegation consists of six permanent delegates and four special delegates. The permanent delegates are appointed by the nine provincial legislatures. The four special delegates consist of the premier of the province and three other special delegates assigned from members of the provincial legislature (https://www.parliament.gov.za/, accessed 13 August 2016).

The executive function of the country is invested in the president, who is elected by the members of the National Assembly. Although each political party puts forward the names of its candidate for president, the candidate of the majority party becomes the president. The national cabinet is made up of ministers and deputy ministers who are appointed by the president. Box 6.1 provides an overview of the electoral system and process in South Africa.

The legislative function of the province is invested in the provincial legislature (parliament). In terms of the Constitution, provinces are responsible for passing legislation in a number of functional areas, which are listed in two schedules (Republic of South Africa, 1996). The executive function of the province is invested in the premier, elected by the members of the provincial legislature. Each political party puts forward the names of its candidate for premier, but in practice the candidate of the majority party becomes the premier. The provincial executive council (or provincial cabinet) is made up of provincial ministers, known as members of the Executive Council (MECs). They are politicians appointed by the premier (often in consultation with the party) and are mandated to implement national policy and functions assigned to the provinces. Provinces can also assign any of these legislative powers to a municipal council if the matter would be most effectively dealt with locally and if the capacity exists to administer it efficiently (Republic of South Africa, 1996).

The powers of the provincial governments are circumscribed by the South African Constitution, which limits them to certain listed functional areas. In some areas the provincial governments' powers are concurrent with those of the national government (e.g., health), while in other areas the national government has exclusive powers (e.g., defence) (Republic of South Africa, 1996).

Box 6.1   Electoral system and process in South Africa

- South Africa is a multiparty democracy and the Constitution is the supreme law of the country.
- Elections are held every five years.
- South Africa uses a proportional representation voting system based on political party lists at the national and provincial levels. A registered political party receives a share of seats in Parliament in direct proportion to the number of votes cast for it in the election.
- Voters don't vote for individuals but for a political party, which decides on members to fill the seats it has won.
- The National Assembly consists of between 350 and 400 seats. Provincial representatives have 50 per cent of seats in the National Assembly and are elected proportionally in each province.
- Members of the National Assembly elect the president from among their members, although each party puts forward the name of its presidential candidate. In practice, the candidate of the majority party becomes the president.
- The National Council of Provinces also participates in legislative processes and was created to ensure cooperative governance and participatory democracy. This body ensures that provincial interests are aligned in national legislation that affects the provinces. The NCOP consists of fifty-four permanent members and thirty-six special delegates.
- Each province is a single constituency for provincial elections.
- By convention the elections of the National Assembly and the provincial legislatures are held at the same time. Members of each provincial legislature elect the premier. As in the case of the National Assembly, each party puts forward the name of its candidate for premier.
- Municipalities are governed by municipal councils. The Municipal Structures Act 1998 introduced a single member (ward), two-tier compensatory proportional system.
- Nationwide municipal elections take place one to two years after national and provincial elections.

Source: http://www.elections.org.za/content/default.aspx/

The Constitution contains rules for resolving conflicts between national and provincial legislation (Republic of South Africa, 1996).

According to section 100(1)(a) of the South African Constitution, the national executive may issue a directive to the provincial executive instructing it to comply with its constitutional and other obligations and stating the steps necessary for it to do so. This is expected to be a collaborative process, with both national and provincial departments working together to remedy the identified problems. Section 100(1)(b) allows the national executive to go further and actually "assume responsibility" for the obligation or place the provincial department "under administration." This can only happen after attempts to resolve the problem under section 100(1)(a) have failed and the provincial executive has not complied with a directive (Republic of South Africa, 1996). For example, in 2012, the South African Cabinet implemented section 100(1)(b) of the Constitution in respect of five departments, including Health, in the Limpopo Province (National Treasury, 2012b). This was a direct intervention by the national executive because the provincial government accumulated unauthorized expenditure of R2.7 billion in the 2011/12 fiscal year and largely ignored the warnings from the National Treasury (National Treasury, 2012b). In the same year, line departments in the Eastern Cape, Free State, and Gauteng were also placed under administration, for reasons that included large amounts of unauthorized expenditure, noncompliance with national legislation, poor supply chain management, and illegal and unfunded contractual commitments (National Treasury, 2012b).

At the local government level, the executive authority is invested in a democratically elected mayor. When a municipality cannot fulfil its function as outlined in the Constitution, the provincial executive may assume responsibility for the relevant obligation, with similar provisions as outlined above (Republic of South Africa, 1996).

Competency for Health

Section 27 of the Constitution contains the Bill of Rights that oblige the government to ensure the rights of all citizens to have access to health care services (including reproductive health services); promote and protect the right of children to basic health care services; and ensure that no one is refused emergency medical treatment (Republic of South Africa, 1996). However, the Constitution allows for "the progressive realization of the right of access to health care services," which means that this right can be implemented over time as the country's fiscal resources permit.

As with general responsibilities, decentralized governance of the health sector is defined by the South African Constitution, which outlines the powers and functions of the three spheres of government (Republic of South Africa, 1996; Van Rensburg, 2004). Health services are listed as a concurrent functional area, and legislation can be passed at both national and provincial levels (Figure 6.2).

The Constitution grants the national level the power to pass national legislation, set norms and standards, relate to international organizations, and monitor the delivery of health care. The Constitution also assigns responsibility to provinces for the planning and delivery (implementation) of services. Although the Constitution grants local government the responsibility for the delivery of municipal health services, these services are defined in the National Health Act (Republic of South Africa, 1996).

By law, the national or provincial governments can delegate authority for concurrent issues, such as health, to local government. However, since provinces have the constitutional responsibility for the delivery of health care services, they are expected to pass provincial legislation to implement and regulate such delivery (Republic of South Africa, 1996). Should a conflict exist between provincial and national health legislation, national legislation takes precedence, provided one or all of the following conditions are met: that the policy issue or problem cannot be effectively regulated at the provincial level, that another province would be prejudiced, or that national security would be undermined (Republic of South Africa, 1996).

The Municipal Systems Act of 2000 gives prominence to two issues, critical for the establishment of the district health system: community participation and integrated development planning (Republic of South Africa, 2000). The Municipal Systems Act advocates for the building of a culture of community participation and imposes an obligation on local government to provide information and mechanisms for community participation to be meaningful. Integrated development planning is an obligation for all municipalities and provides the opportunity for intersectoral action at the local government level, and for local government departments (such as health, water, and sanitation and public works) to align their infrastructural and development needs into a common framework to ensure effective, long-term development (Republic of South Africa, 2000).

Health Care Financing

In South Africa, 8.6 per cent of the gross domestic product (GDP) is spent on health care, and government spending on health care is 4.2 per cent (Blecher, Kollipara, de Jager, & Zulu, 2011). Although spending on the public health sector has doubled in real terms over the past fifteen years, government spending remains at around 41.4 per cent of total health care spending due to similar growth in private health expenditure (Blecher et al., 2011). The private health

Figure 6.2 Political organization of the South African health system

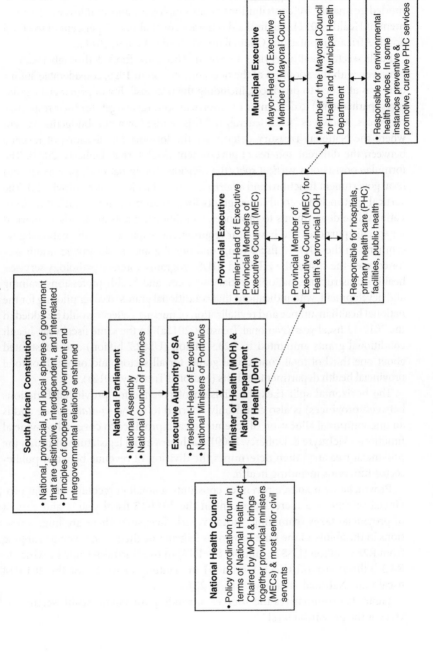

South African Constitution
• National, provincial, and local spheres of government that are distinctive, interdependent, and interrelated
• Principles of cooperative government and intergovernmental relations enshrined

National Parliament
• National Assembly
• National Council of Provinces

Executive Authority of SA
• President-Head of Executive
• National Ministers of Portfolios

Minister of Health (MOH) & National Department of Health (DoH)

National Health Council
• Policy coordination forum in terms of National Health Act Chaired by MOH & brings together provincial ministers (MECs) & most senior civil servants

Provincial Executive
• Premier-Head of Executive
• Provincial Members of Executive Council (MEC)

• Provincial Member of Executive Council (MEC) for Health & provincial DOH

• Responsible for hospitals, primary health care (PHC) facilities, public health

Municipal Executive
• Mayor-Head of Executive
• Member of Mayoral Council

• Member of the Mayoral Council for Health and Municipal Health Department

• Responsible for environmental health services. In some instances preventive & promotive, curative PHC services

sector is dominated by private health insurance (called medical aid schemes), funded primarily by contributions from employers and employees (Department of Health, 2011). Medical aid schemes cover about 17 per cent of the total South African population (Council for Medical Schemes, 2011).

Public-sector health services in South Africa are funded through taxation. However, with the adoption of the new constitution in 1996, considerable autonomy was afforded to provinces, including the responsibility of provincial legislatures (parliaments) to determine functional or sectoral budgets for their respective provinces. Known as "fiscal federalism," this resulted in a new budgeting system where the National Treasury determines the formula for divisions of revenue between the different spheres of government (McIntyre & Doherty, 2009). The formula consists of a *vertical split* (the division among national, provincial, and local government function) and a *horizontal split* (block grants to provinces). The vertical split includes conditional grants for certain programs, which flow from national line departments to provinces. Conditional grants are funds earmarked for specific purposes and have clear requirements stipulated by the national government. In the 2011/12 fiscal year, conditional grants to the public health sector covered the cost of the HIV and AIDS programs, forensic pathology services, health infrastructure, national tertiary services, and health professions training and development, with indications that conditional grants to cover piloting for the national health insurance and revitalization of nursing colleges would be added in the 2012/13 fiscal year (National Treasury, 2012a). In the same fiscal year, health conditional grants amounted to R23.9 billion (US$2.7 billion) and constituted about one-third of total conditional grants for all sectors and one-fifth of total provincial health department budgets (National Treasury, 2012a).

The horizontal split (i.e., the division of revenue for provincial functions between provinces) is also commonly referred to as the *equitable share* and is an unconditional allocation of revenue to each province to cover all provincial functions (McIntyre & Doherty, 2009). Each provincial legislature (through the provincial treasury) then determines the division of revenue between public-sector functions including health.

Provincial own-source revenues constitute a small percentage of total provincial revenue – a mere 3 per cent in the 2014/15 fiscal year – and consist of provincial taxes (gambling, motor vehicle licenses). There are huge variations in the ability of the nine provinces to generate their own revenue, ranging from R283 million (US$21 million; $1=R13) in the Northern Cape Province to R4.3 billion (around US$331 million) in Gauteng Province for the 2013/14 fiscal year (National Treasury, 2015, p. 22).

Figure 6.3 summarizes the sources of funding for public health sector services at the provincial level.

Figure 6.3 Sources of provincial public health sector funding

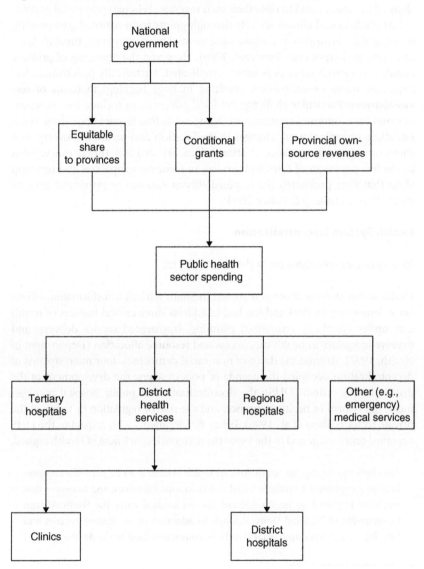

Municipalities are entitled, in terms of the Constitution, to an equitable share of tax money and to raise their own revenue. Whereas provincial governments are financed almost entirely through grants from national government, municipal governments as a whole raise most of their own funds through taxes and service charges (van Ryneveld, 2006). However, the financing of primary health care (PHC) services is more complicated. Historically government has neglected many municipalities, resulting in huge backlogs in terms of service delivery. Particular challenges of local government include the increased demand for economic infrastructure; aging assets that require upgrading, rehabilitation, or replacement; changes in the location and nature of poverty; and shortcomings in governance (National Treasury, 2012a). This is exacerbated by the low payments of rates and services in some municipalities and function shifts that were previously the responsibility of national or provincial governments (Van Rensburg & Pelser, 2004).

Health System Decentralization

History of Decentralization in the Health Sector

Health sector decentralization is rooted in South Africa's transformation efforts since democracy in 1994 and has had to address three critical features of health care under apartheid: centralized planning, fragmented service delivery, and massive inequities in health care access and resource allocation (Department of Health, 1997). Around the dawn of non-racial democracy, four main streams of decentralization occupied the agenda of policymakers: the development of the district health system (DHS); the decentralization of public hospital management; the reform of health insurance; and the role of regulation in terms of the private sector (Gilson et al., 1996). Policy developments with respect to the DHS occupied centre stage and in the 1990s the national Department of Health argued,

> The challenge facing the South African health system is to be part of a comprehensive programme to redress social and economic injustices, and to ensure that emphasis is placed on health and not just on medical care. The South African Government of National Unity, through its adoption of the Reconstruction and Development Programme (RDP)[2] in 1994, committed itself to the development of

---

2 The RDP was an integrated, coherent socio-economic policy framework outlining strategies to reduce poverty and address the huge shortfall and disparities in the provision of social services in South Africa which existed in 1994. Many of proposals contained in the document found their way into government policies and legislation.

a District Health System based on the Primary Health Care Approach as enunci-
ated at Alma Ata in 1978. (Department of Health, 1995, p. 1)

The Policy for the Development of a District Health System for South Africa
was released in 1995 to guide the implementation of the DHS (Department of
Health & Health Policy Coordinating Unit, 1995). In 1997, the *White Paper
for the Transformation of the Health System in South Africa* outlined a set of
policy objectives and principles upon which a unified national health system
would be based (Department of Health, 1997). The white paper proposed the
establishment of a DHS that would ensure the delivery of comprehensive PHC
(Department of Health, 1997). The PHC approach, a philosophical approach
outlined in the 1978 World Health Organization (WHO) Alma-Ata Declaration, was seen as the "most effective and cost effective means of improving
the population's health" (Department of Health, 1997). The 1997 white paper
outlined a wide range of PHC services provided as ambulatory care services
outside hospitals. These services included personal promotive and preventive
services (such as health education, family planning, and immunization); personal curative services for acute minor ailments; minor trauma; maternal and
child health such as antenatal care and uncomplicated deliveries; provision of
essential drugs; and basic rehabilitation services, all supported by a network of
referral services (Department of Health, 1997).

The 1997 white paper proposed three governance options for the DHS:

1. *Provincial option.* The province would be responsible for all district health
services through a district health manager. This option would apply to those
situations where there is insufficient capacity and infrastructure at the local
government level.

2. *Statutory district health authority option.* The province, through legislation, would create a district health authority for each health district. This option would apply in those circumstances where no single local authority had
the capacity to render comprehensive PHC services.

3. *Local government option.* A local authority would be responsible for
all district health services. This option would apply in those instances where
the local authority had the capacity to render comprehensive PHC services.
(Department of Health, 1997)

Each of these options had different funding, policy, and accountability implications. However, regardless of the governance option, it was envisaged that a
health district would be responsible for the overall management of all health
care services within its jurisdiction; ensure collaboration between the private,

public, and non-governmental sectors; be responsible and accountable for its own budget; and provide, or purchase, a comprehensive range of primary health care services.

All policy documents since 1994 have highlighted the need to have health districts aligned with political and administrative boundaries, and this was achieved by 2001 (Barron & Asia, 2001).

However, the delay in finalizing national legislation to provide legal certainty around the structure and functioning of the DHS was a major constraint to health system decentralization (Harrison & Qose, 1998; Van Rensburg & Pelser, 2004). In 1998, it was pointed out that the national Department of Health faced "the unenviable task of establishing a legislative framework for the national health system without impinging on the constitutional integrity of provincial and local spheres of government" (Harrison & Qose, 1998, p. 23).

This legislative vacuum presented numerous implementation challenges (Van Rensburg & Pelser, 2004). Progress in integrating the primary health care services provided by provincial and local government was slow, especially in metropolitan areas (such as Johannesburg and Cape Town). The already sensitive relationship between local government and provincial departments of health was exacerbated by different conditions of service, lack of clarity on resource allocation, and lack of clarity on the definition of municipal health services (Van Rensburg & Pelser, 2004). Notwithstanding the potential benefits of decentralization, numerous health analysts stressed the importance of achieving equity in health care delivery within and between provinces, and of overcoming the historical fragmentation of service delivery (Harrison & Qose, 1998; Van Rensburg & Pelser, 2004).

In 2001, a number of milestones were reached with regard to the development of the DHS (Barron & Asia, 2001). The Health MINMEC[3] (Minister and Members of the Executive Councils), an intergovernmental advisory forum made up of the national health minister, the provincial health ministers, and senior civil servants in the national and provincial health departments, endorsed the vision of a municipality-based DHS in South Africa (Barron & Asia, 2001). Other key decisions included the following:

- District and metropolitan council areas shall be the focal point for the organization and coordination of health services.
- Provincial departments of health will be responsible for coordinating, planning, and delivery of health services within these areas, in collaboration with local government.

---

3 The Health MINMEC is now called the National Health Council, which remains an advisory, intergovernmental forum.

- Each MEC for Health (provincial minister) shall establish a provincial health authority and facilitate the establishment of a district health authority (DHA).
- Municipalities should have the capacity to deliver comprehensive PHC services (but these services would exclude district hospitals).
- After conducting an audit of health services, the MEC for Health may delegate the delivery of health services to the metropolitan or district council, with the appropriate capacity, support, and resources. The relationship would be managed by a service-level agreement between the province and the municipality with clearly outlined performance indicators. (Barron & Asia, 2001)

In the absence of a national legislative framework for DHS development, many provinces developed their own legislation, policies, and implementation strategies (Barron & Asia, 2001). The provincial acts varied in content and presentation, but all made some legislative commitment to the DHS and the decentralization of health to local government, using terms such as "delegate, assign, transfer and/or devolve" health services to local government (HST, 2002). In addition to defining the DHS, by 2001, six out of nine provinces had established provincial health authorities (Barron & Asia, 2001).

In November 2001, the National Health Bill was published for public comment (Barron & Asia, 2001). In an attempt to protect the revenue that the large metropolitan councils spent on health, the definition of municipal health services was left vague on purpose, exacerbating the confusion of roles, duplication, and fragmentation between the provinces and the local authorities that already existed (Barron & Asia, 2001).

However, in order to finalize national health legislation, the Health MINMEC was obliged to adopt a much narrower definition of municipal health services (Van Rensburg & Pelser, 2004). In terms of the 2003 National Health Act, *municipal health services* are defined as water quality management, food control, waste management, health surveillance of premises, prevention of communicable diseases (excluding immunizations), vector control, environmental pollution control, disposal of the dead, and chemical safety (Republic of South Africa, 2004). The vision of local government assuming responsibility for a full package of health services (including district hospitals) remained among national and provincial health stakeholders. It was envisaged that provincial governments would delegate, through service-level agreements and with the necessary resources, other PHC services to a district or metropolitan municipality where the capacity existed (Van Rensburg & Pelser, 2004).

The National Health Act (Act 61 of 2003), eventually promulgated in 2005, provides the legislative framework for the delivery of health care services and puts into effect the vision set out in the *White Paper on the Transformation of the Health System* (Republic of South Africa, 2004). The act sets out the structures, mechanisms, resources, and systems aimed at the progressive realization (i.e., over time) of every citizen's right of access to health care services.

Under the National Health Act, the National Health Council replaced the Health MINMEC, although the composition of the structure remains unchanged. At a provincial level, provincial health councils and consultative bodies were created and the DHS was established (Republic of South Africa, 2004). The MEC for Health may subdivide any district into sub-districts and establish a district health council, the functions of which are to promote cooperative governance; ensure the coordination of planning, budgeting, provisioning, and monitoring of all health services that affect residents of the health district for which the council was established; and advise the MEC, through a provincial health council, and the municipal council, on any matter regarding health or health services in the health district (Republic of South Africa, 2004).

The act outlines the functions of the national and provincial departments of health (Republic of South Africa, 2004). Districts may be subdivided into sub-districts in consultation with local government. The establishment of district health councils is the responsibility of the MEC for Health, and the district health council must include representation from both province and local government. Provincial legislation must provide for the functioning of district councils (Republic of South Africa, 2004).

Since 2013, the DHS, decentralization, and appropriate governance structures (e.g., independent DHAs) have been under review, motivated by the proposed reforms contained in the 2011 *Green Paper on National Health Insurance* (Department of Health, 2011) and its successor, the *White Paper on National Health Insurance in South Africa* (Department of Health, 2015). The stated objectives of the National Health Insurance (NHI) reforms are as follows: to improve access to quality services; to pool risks and funds to achieve equity and social solidarity; to mobilize and control key financial resources in an efficient manner; and to improve health sector performance (Department of Health, 2011; Department of Health, 2015). Recognizing the complexity of the proposals and that many technical, operational, and financial aspects require further details (National Treasury, 2012a), the national government proposed that the NHI be implemented over a fourteen-year period, with the first five years focusing on strengthening the government health sector.

The NHI proposals envisage a purchaser/provider split. The strengthening of PHC will be a focus of the NHI during the first five-year phase. Although the 2011 green paper proposed that DHAs will be the main "contracting units," supported by the subnational offices of the NHI fund (Department of Health, 2011), there is no mention of DHAs in the white paper (Department of Health, 2015).

In contrast, the white paper has proposed the establishment of district health management offices (DHMOs) to manage district health services. It suggests that the "DHMOs will be structures to which management, planning and coordination of personal and non-personal health service provision responsibilities are delegated, taking into account national health policy priorities and guidelines as well as health needs in the district" (Department of Health, 2015, p. 35).

In the 2012/13 fiscal year, pilot sites were established in selected districts to begin laying the foundations of the NHI, namely improved facilities, skilled managers, and re-engineering of PHC. The Treasury established a new conditional grant for these pilot projects in the 2012 budget, with allocations amounting to R150 million in fiscal year 1 (US$11.5 million), R350 million (US$26.9 million) in fiscal year 2, and R500 million (US$38.5 million) in fiscal year 3 (National Treasury, 2012a). The pilot projects were aimed to provide practical lessons on new models for PHC services, including municipal-based PHC services, district clinical support teams, and school health services (National Treasury, 2012a).

At the same time, the NHI proposals are silent on the role of provincial health departments. The proposed DHMOs are evolving and are the subject of a separate NHI task team (work stream). However, there is no clarity in the white paper on the links of these proposed structures to provincial health departments and to the current district health system.

Decentralization to Districts: Progress and Challenges

The National Health Act provides the legislative framework for a decentralized DHS in South Africa. A functional DHS is expected to ensure the delivery of quality, equitable PHC services as envisaged at Alma-Ata (WHO, 1978), improve health outcomes for all South Africans (Department of Health, 2010), and change the power relations between the centre (province) and the periphery (district) (Van Rensburg & Pelser, 2004). However, in practice, the lack of clarity on the roles and responsibilities of the different levels of government has led to a more confused picture.

Some progress has occurred along the act's prescriptions. All provinces have established districts, and the district boundaries are coterminous with municipal boundaries. In many instances, provinces have established sub-districts serving a population of between 150,000 and 300,000 people.

District health management teams have also been established and many managers have undergone training. Some decentralization of decision-making and authority has also taken place (Development Bank of South Africa, 2008; HST, 2008).

However, overall progress with the implementation of the National Health Act has been slow (Rispel & Moorman, 2010). Only one province has passed legislation to establish district health councils; hence most health districts do not function as envisaged in the National Health Act. There have also been several constraints on the establishment of district health systems, including tension and lack of trust between provinces and their local governments because of funding and capacity problems, uncertainty regarding the flow of funding and the role of the provinces or district hospitals in the case of a local government model, and ineffective and inefficient management systems (Van Rensburg & Pelser, 2004). Importantly, the role of local government in the delivery of PHC has changed. Although the Health MINMEC resolved in 2001 that PHC will fall under local government, by 2005, the National Health Council resolved that PHC should be a provincial responsibility. This was in part due to funding constraints, perceived loss of control by the provincial health departments, and tension between provincial and local government health department staff. In response to this resolution, all municipal clinics were to be transferred to provincial health structures, a process known as provincialization. But the process of provincialization has been messy and remains incomplete. In metropolitan municipalities, both provincial and local government health departments continue to employ staff and render PHC services, and in some areas, provincial departments of health deliver PHC services through infrastructure owned by local governments.

The constitutional autonomy of provincial departments of health creates the conditions for different interpretations of what constitutes a DHS and what structures and mechanisms are most appropriate to ensure implementation (Integrated Support Teams, 2009; Van Rensburg, 2004). Marked variations emerged, exacerbated by human resource constraints and suboptimal stewardship and leadership from the national level (Coovadia, Jewkes, Barron, Sanders, & McIntyre, 2009; Rispel & Setswe, 2007).

Importantly, these districts are not functioning as originally intended (Naledi, Barron, & Schneider, 2011). Although the districts have district health management teams responsible for the day-to-day management of PHC facilities, they are not functioning as management entities with delegated authority. The districts are not statutory bodies with fully delegated authority and budgets; they are, in reality, deconcentrated units reporting to the provincial health authority. The extent of the delegations varies considerably across and within provinces (Integrated Support Teams, 2009). There are notable differences in the financial delegations, with the maximum amount that district managers may authorize ranging from R5,000 (US$385) in the Northern Cape Province to R1 million (US$76,923) in the Eastern Cape Province. In terms of the Public Finance Management Act (PFMA), the head of the provincial department of health remains the accounting officer (Republic of South Africa, 1999). Without the appropriate delegations, district managers cannot make decisions, and the perceived benefits of decentralization – namely accountability to communities, improved health outcomes, and access to quality services – have not been realized.

There is also a lack of uniformity in the composition of district health management teams both between and within provinces, reflected in highly variable expenditure on the district management function, ranging from 0.6 per cent to 28.1 per cent of district health budgets in 2006/7 (Day, Barron, Monticelli, & Sello, 2009). The sub-district level, which conforms more closely to the WHO notion of the ideal district of 150,000 to 300,000 people and where much of the decision-making on PHC should ultimately reside, is even less developed.

Human resources delegations in particular are very limited, with almost none of the district managers able to control staff establishments or approve the hiring and firing of staff. Some of the limitations in delegations are due to a lack of guidance from national level, a lack of management capacity, high turnover of staff, and high vacancy rates at the district level (Development Bank of South Africa, 2008; Integrated Support Teams, 2009). In addition, district hospitals still function separately from and are poorly coordinated with PHC services in many places, and formal mechanisms of accountability such as district councils and clinic/community health centre committees are either absent or not playing a meaningful role. At the same time, improving the functionality and management of the health system is a priority for the national government. The 2012/13 Annual Performance Plan indicates an intention to review the delegations to hospital and district managers to ensure competent health management and to implement appropriately decentralized and accountable management in all fifty-two districts (Department of Health, 2012).

In 2012, the national minister of health launched ten pilot projects to assess various policy options for the NHI. Conditional grant funding totalling R1.3 billion (US$100 million) over three years provides financial support to the pilot projects, which have been established in all provinces and cover about ten million people (National Treasury, 2013). Although the minister of health has provided visible leadership on the current set of ambitious health care reforms, there has been insufficient consultation with (and buy-in from) the provinces, whose authority has been challenged by the direct management and intervention of the national health department in the pilot NHI districts

(Rispel & Moorman, 2013). Only time will tell whether these reforms, even though accompanied by strong political stewardship, will result in significant decentralization and its intended health service benefits.

Decision Space in the South African Health System

This section uses Bossert's 1998 framework of decision space (Bossert, 1998), a review of existing literature, and the authors' own experience of the South African health system to judge whether the relevant actor (provincial health department, public hospitals, or districts) has narrow, moderate, or broad authority in exercising its health system responsibilities. First, the decision space between the national and provincial health departments is examined (Table 6.1).

As can be seen in Table 6.1, the provincial health departments are financed almost entirely through grants from the national government, which could make the decision space narrow in terms of Bossert's framework. However, the provincial health departments have considerable autonomy, as health is a concurrent jurisdiction in the Constitution (Republic of South Africa, 1996) and the bulk of the grants from the national government are block grants with no conditions. In 2009, an assessment of the performance of the health system found that there were ten de facto health departments in operation in South Africa (Integrated Support Teams, 2009). The system of fiscal federalism in South Africa means that the national Department of Health has little say over provincial governments' funding for health, except through the conditional grants, which constitute around one-fifth of provincial health budgets. These conditional grants are the principal means used by the national government to set national standards and achieve national health system objectives (McIntyre & Doherty, 2009). At the same time, there have been suboptimal financial management, reporting, and accountability processes for the conditional grants, with minimal or no consequences for the errant provincial health departments (Integrated Support Teams, 2009). Although a national coordinating mechanism determines user fees, provincial health departments can raise funds through hospital user fees (PHC services are free at the point of contact), and hence the decision space could be judged as moderate.

With regard to governance, although the hospital boards are prescribed in the National Health Act (Republic of South Africa, 2004), there are no rules about the size, number, or composition of the provincial health department or the district offices. The only limit is the budget. One of the consequences is the inadequate structural linkages, coordination, and communication between the national and the provincial health departments (Integrated Support Teams, 2009). The National Health Act provides an enabling framework for community

Table 6.1 Provincial health department decision space in South Africa (hospital and primary health care services)

Function	Indicator	Range of Choice		
		Narrow	Moderate	Wide
Financing				
Sources of revenue	Intergovernmental transfers as % of provincial health spending		Receive bulk of funding from national government, but these are unrestricted	
Allocation of expenditures	% of provincial spending that is explicitly earmarked by national health authorities		Earmarking for some national tertiary services, health professional training, hospital priorities, and some national norms and standards, but major funding is unrestricted	
Income from fees and contracts	Extent to which provincial governments can raise funds through user fees for hospital services		PHC services are free; a uniform patient fee schedule for hospitals determined through national coordinating process with provincial health participation	
Service organization and delivery				
Hospital autonomy	Range of autonomy for hospitals	Prescribed by law		
Payment mechanisms	Choice of how providers (hospitals and PHC facilities) paid (incentives and non-salaried)	Prescribed by law		
Physician autonomy	Choice of how physicians governed, organized, and paid	Prescribed by law		
Required programs	Specificity of norms for provincial programs		National guidelines available for some programs (e.g., TB, HIV & AIDS)	
Human resources				
Salaries	Choice of salary range	Prescribed by Public Service Act and central bargaining		

(Continued)

Table 6.1 Provincial health department decision space in South Africa (hospital and primary health care services) (Conitnued)

Function	Indicator	Range of Choice		
		Narrow	Moderate	Wide
Human resources				
Contracting Civil service	Contracting non-permanent staff Hiring and firing of permanent staff	Prescribed by Labour Relations Act Prescribed by Public Service and Labour Relations Acts		
Access rules				
Targeting	Defining priority populations	Constitution makes provision for universal access, although some prioritization of certain groups can happen at provincial level		
Governance rules				
Provincial health administration	National rules limiting size, number, or composition of provincial health department			No limits, except the budget
District offices	Size and composition of local offices			No limits, except budget
Facility (hospital) boards	Size and composition of boards	Prescribed in terms of National Health Act; minister appoints boards of central hospitals, provincial ministers appoint boards of all other hospitals		
Community participation	Size, number, composition, and role of community participation		National Health Act states that the most senior civil servants at national and provincial health departments must promote community participation in the planning, provision, and evaluation of health services	

participation, and the provinces have a broad space for potential engagement with civil society. Access rules are enshrined in the South African Constitution. The state must protect, promote, and fulfil the rights enshrined in the Bill of Rights, a cornerstone of democracy in South Africa. In terms of section 27 of the Constitution, the state must take reasonable legislative and other measures within its available resources to achieve the progressive realization of the right of the people of South Africa to have access to health care services (Republic of South Africa, 1996). No one may be refused emergency medical treatment, every child has the right to basic health care services, and everyone has the right to live and work in an environment that is not harmful to their health or well-being (Republic of South Africa, 1996).

In the first five years of democracy, access to health care was extended, especially to those without prior access (African National Congress, 1994). Informed by the constitutional provision, which stipulates children's rights to basic nutrition, shelter, basic health care services, and social services (Republic of South Africa, 1996), the emphasis on increasing access to health care in the first term of governance was underlined in the presidential address to Parliament on 24 May 1994, when Nelson Mandela declared the policy of free health care for children under the age of six, for pregnant women, and for women in the postnatal period. This free health care policy was implemented within the first one hundred days of democratic government (McCoy, 1996). All PHC services subsequently became free, and health services at all levels of facilities are also free for certain categories (e.g., pensioners, persons receiving social grants or with disabilities) and for certain services (e.g., tuberculosis management, voluntary counselling and testing for HIV, medico-legal services for survivors of sexual assault). Children and pregnant women covered by private medical insurance or living in households that earn more than R100,000 (US$7,692) per year are not eligible for free health care (Republic of South Africa, 2004).

Human resources rules are governed by the national Department of Public Service and Administration (DPSA). The DPSA provides guidelines on organizational design, post establishment, job evaluation, performance management, and compensation of employees (Integrated Support Teams, 2009). The national Department of Health focuses on the overall planning and provision of trained health professionals and provides strategies, plans, and guidelines of national concern, such as the nursing strategy, national human resources for health planning framework, rural retention strategy, foreign doctors policy, and interaction with and ensuring capacity of tertiary and academic training institutions – in collaboration with the Department of Education (Integrated Support Teams, 2009). Although provinces are largely autonomous and implement the various acts, regulations, and guidelines according to their own situation and requirements (Integrated Support Teams, 2009), the decision space is prescribed by law and therefore narrow.

The decision space for service delivery and organization is also relatively narrow and prescribed by public-sector legislation. National norms, standards, and guidelines are not available in many areas, and where these are available, implementation is suboptimal and varies considerably across the nine provinces. This is exacerbated by fragmented planning processes both within the national Department of Health and between the department and the provinces (Integrated Support Teams, 2009).

The decision space is even narrower when the framework is applied to public hospitals and districts in the key functional areas (Table 6.2). Until recently, analysts have suggested that bureaucratic inertia, incompetence, and a lack of political will contributed to the absence of the meaningful delegation of authority and accountability to public hospitals and district offices (Development Bank of South Africa, 2008). In 2013, developments in increasing decentralization to public hospitals included the publication of regulations on designation (categorization) of hospitals, services to be provided by each category of hospital, and policy on their management. It is envisaged that the regulations will be "a key step in ensuring the appointment of competent and skilled managers, the decentralisation of management and the development of accountability frameworks" (Matsoso & Fryatt, 2013, p. 22). In addition, there has been a concerted effort to place strong managers as CEOs of selected hospitals.

Health System Capacity of Provincial Governments

Notwithstanding the constitutional provisions of concurrency for health, the decision space authority of provincial health departments ranges from narrow to broad. The reasons for this variation are complex but influenced by issues at both national and provincial government levels. Historically, the national health department has provided insufficient leadership and stewardship to ensure that available health resources are commensurate with a range of national policies and the requirements needed for implementation (Integrated Support Teams, 2009). A 2009 health system assessment found material unfunded mandates arising from pressures on the allocated budget beyond the control of the most senior civil servants, namely the heads of departments who are accountable for aligning expenditure to allocated budgets (Integrated Support Teams, 2009). In 2009, unfunded mandates included the following: a civil service financial incentive known as occupation-specific dispensation that was not fully budgeted; new vaccines that were insufficiently funded; legislative requirements such as the creation of the district health system; the

Table 6.2 Public hospitals and health district decision space for the administration and delivery of publicly funded health services

Function	Indicator	Range of Choice		
		Narrow	Moderate	Wide
Financing				
Source of revenue	Provincial funding as a % of hospital and district office spending	Almost 100% of revenues from provincial governments		
Expenditure allocation	% of spending explicitly earmarked by provincial government	Salary and capital spending set by provincial government, with limits on amount of money that can be moved between programs		
Fees	Extent to which hospitals can raise revenues through fees for services	Uniform national patient fee schedule		
Procurement	Extent to which hospitals or districts can set own procurement rules	Governed by national laws		
Service organization and delivery				
Required programs	Rules on what services must be delivered	Set by provincial government		
Hospital autonomy	Choice of how hospitals governed, organized, and paid	Provincial government		
Human resources				
Salaries	Choice of salary range	Prescribed by Public Service Act and central bargaining		
Contracting	Contracting non-permanent staff	Prescribed by Labour Relations Act		
Civil service	Hiring and firing of permanent staff	Prescribed by Public Service and Labour Relations Acts		

(Continued)

Table 6.2 Public hospitals and health district decision space for the administration and delivery of publicly funded health services (Continued)

Function	Indicator	Range of Choice		
		Narrow	Moderate	Wide
Access rules				
Targeting	Extent to which subpopulations or services can be targeted	Constitution makes provision for universal access, although some prioritization of certain groups can happen at provincial level		
Population served	Extent to which district can determine whether it should provide services to individuals not resident within its boundaries	National and provincial government sets policy in terms of services		
Governance rules				
Hospital board appointment	Degree to which board members elected by public or appointed by provincial minister	Board members appointed by provincial health minister, central hospital boards appointed by national minister		
Mandate	Degree to which hospital or district can set own mandate, or if provincially set, the flexibility of mandate	Has to comply with national and provincial laws, policies and strategies		

takeover of local government functions and staff that were not funded; and political promises made by provincial ministers, such as the building of new clinics (Integrated Support Teams, 2009). Planning processes were also fragmented both within the national Department of Health and between national and provincial departments of health, resulting in some contradictions in service norms and standards for key health priority programs (Integrated Support Teams, 2009).

At the provincial level, instability in senior management and in administrative and human resource capacity has influenced the ability of provincial health departments to exercise their decision-making authority. The government's own statistics have shown that within a sample of eleven departments there was almost a 30 per cent turnover among senior managers (Public Service Commission, 2011). Those provincial health departments (such as the Western Cape and KwaZulu Natal) that enjoyed some continuity in senior management have exercised a greater decision-making capacity than those where there has been a high turnover. Gauteng Province, the economic powerhouse of the country, has had a high turnover of provincial health ministers, with the third one governing since the 2009 elections. Similarly, there have been four different provincial heads of health between 2009 and 2014.

Administrative and human resource capacity also varies greatly across the nine provinces (Rispel, de Jager, & Fonn, 2016; Rispel & Moorman, 2013). In the 2010/11 fiscal year, the majority (78 per cent) of these provincial health departments received either a qualified or adverse audit outcome for the financial year (Auditor-General of South Africa, 2011). In addition, the auditor-general found the majority of provinces showed weaknesses in the implementation of health information systems (seven of nine), that reports on HIV statistics were unreliable (seven of nine), that ambulance staff or vehicles were not available (seven of nine), and that new clinics or health facilities were either unutilized or underutilized (six of nine) (Auditor-General of South Africa, 2011). The National Planning Commission also pointed to problems in provincial administrative capacity, resulting in "poor authority, feeble accountability, marginalisation of clinical processes and low staff morale" (National Planning Commission, 2011, p. 301).

As indicated earlier, in 2012, the South African Cabinet placed the Eastern Cape, Free State, Gauteng, and Limpopo under administration (National Treasury, 2012b). In 2013, a Treasury budget review notes that "service delivery in certain areas has fallen short of expectations due to lack of effective planning, inadequate state capacity and the absence of clear lines of responsibility" (National Treasury, 2013, p. 4).

Culture of Federalism in South Africa

Notwithstanding the existence of legislated structures for intergovernmental relations, a 2009 health systems assessment found that accountability mechanisms between national and provincial health departments were deficient (Integrated Support Teams, 2009). In practice, the national health department depended on the provincial health departments to achieve national health goals and policies (Integrated Support Teams, 2009). Provincial respondents believed that national policies were not followed up or supported during implementation at the provincial level. Although national policies contain the core strategies, these lack clear guidelines on implementation, further complicated by unclear roles and responsibilities between different levels of management (Integrated Support Teams, 2009).

Projected overspending in provincial health departments is often accompanied by the withdrawal of delegation of authority from hospitals and district offices. This means that provincial head offices assume responsibility for operational management of health facilities, leading to widespread feelings of disempowerment and lack of accountability within health facilities (Integrated Support Teams, 2009). Many of these issues have not been resolved, and the lack of a fully functional district health system remains one of the major fault lines of health sector transformation in South Africa (Rispel, 2016).

Trends and Conclusions

This chapter set out to analyse health system decentralization in South Africa, focusing on divisions of competencies, funding mechanisms, and means of cooperation between different levels of government to ensure equity, access, quality, and efficiency of health care in a federal political system. The key issues emerging from the analysis are summarized in Box 6.2.

Health system decentralization is enshrined in the Reconstruction and Development Program, the South African Constitution, the *White Paper on the Transformation of the Health System*, and the National Health Act. Much of the first five years of democracy (1994–9) focused on transforming the legacy of apartheid health services, based on PHC principles delivered through well-functioning district health systems. The essence of the DHS was described in the *White Paper for the Transformation of the Health System in South Africa* in 1997 (Department of Health, 1997). It was clear that the envisaged DHS focused on principles including overcoming fragmentation, equity, quality, access to services, local accountability, community participation, and decentralization. The period was characterized by legislative, policy, and structural

---

Box 6.2   Key review findings on health system decentralization in South Africa

1. There is an enabling legal and policy framework that facilitates health system decentralization.
2. Progress on transforming the legacy of apartheid health services includes policy and legislative changes, structural changes to overcome fragmentation, improved access to primary health care services, and resource redistribution.
3. There are different conceptual phases in the policy development and approach to health system decentralization which roughly correspond to the periods of democratic governance.
4. National health ministerial initiatives between 2012 and 2016 indicate recentralizing tendencies that constrain provincial managerial authority.
5. The constitutional autonomy of provinces creates conditions for different interpretations and non-uniformity of national laws and policies.
6. The notion of decision space authority is not straightforward because of concurrent health jurisdiction and large health grants without conditions.
7. Delegations vary considerably, with narrowest in management functions, broadest in community participation.
8. The reality of implementation at district health system and hospital levels suggests that the health care system remains largely centralized at the national and provincial levels, with little decision-making power at district offices and health facilities (hospitals or health centres).
9. Local government operates independently of provincial and national government, and has not been considered in current health care reforms.
10. There has been reluctance on the part of provinces to decentralize to lower levels and there is limited capacity of some local governments to accept this responsibility.

---

changes to overcome fragmentation and apartheid inequities and to improve access to primary health care services and resource redistribution, both among provinces and within them. A major achievement of this period was the institutionalization of the DHS (and hence decentralization), not only in policies but also in the minds and actions of civil servants responsible for implementing these policies. Unity and the notion of one national health system were important; good cooperation was evident among national, provincial, and local governments, characterized by numerous intergovernmental structures and meetings to develop and shape policy around the DHS. Many of the civil servants at different levels of government had come from anti-apartheid organizations and spoke the same language of transformation. This culminated in the first drafts of the National Health Act. As indicated, these first drafts purposively left the definition of municipal health services vague.

The second and third periods of democratic governance (1999–2009) can be described broadly as the period of implementation or making things work. Although progress was made, this phase was characterized by recognition of implementation's difficulties and managing a federal system. A culture of federalism set in because the constitutional independence of provinces implies that provinces can interpret implementation of such national laws or policies in their own way, as long as they stay within a broad national framework. In reality, the provincial ministers of health are accountable to the provincial premier rather than to the national minister of health. The premiers appoint provincial heads of health departments, who in turn are accountable to the provincial health ministers. The culture of federalism was further entrenched by the suboptimal stewardship of the then national minister of health, who was embroiled in the controversy of AIDS denialism. Furthermore, the 1999 PFMA and inadequate health information systems mitigated against decentralization to districts and hospitals, as the provincial head of health is the accounting officer, hence by law accountable for all matters pertaining to financial management. Heads of both district offices and hospitals are designated responsibility officers, but should anything go wrong, the provincial head of health would be answerable.

The period since the 2009 elections has seen recognition of the need for stronger national leadership and stewardship and for regaining health policy and implementation control. Many have realized that PHC and district health systems have not been prioritized sufficiently, that the management and performance of the district health system have been suboptimal, and that the national ministry had to overcome the fragmentation caused by provincial health federalism. This period has been characterized by a revival of PHC, the proposals on the NHI, and a much stronger hand of the national Department of Health in implementation at the district health system and hospital levels (Rispel & Moorman, 2013). The numerous initiatives driven directly by the national ministry and that bypass provincial health departments suggest a recentralizing tendency. Centralizing tendencies constrain provincial managerial authority. An example is the appointment of hospital CEOs in January 2013 in certain provinces by the minister rather than the provincial health departments. However, at the same time, some provincial health departments, particularly where there has been continuity of senior civil servant management, continue to exercise much broader decision space authority. In essence, the health care system remains centralized at the national or provincial level and little decision-making power lies with districts and facilities.

Not surprisingly, provinces have been reluctant to decentralize to local government, and some local governments have been reluctant or have limited capacity to accept this responsibility. In large cities, where there has been an expectation (and some capacity) to assume broader responsibility for PHC services, tensions remain. In some provinces, these metropolitan health departments continue to expand the building of clinics and the provision of an increased range of ambulatory care services. At the same time, the provinces with large cities have moved to regain control of PHC services but have been constrained by lack of funding.

Importantly, decentralization and appropriate governance structures (such as independent district health authorities) are once again on the policy agenda of political decision makers, spearheaded by the proposed NHI system. These health sector reforms present a major opportunity to make decentralization a reality after more than twenty years of democratic governance. At the same time, careful attention needs to be paid to the process of implementation and to change management, thereby ensuring that the vision of broader health sector transformation is not bedevilled by passive resistance and opposition from a powerful provincial lobby and front-line staff, who may have insufficient understanding of these reforms. Successful decentralization requires staff buy-in to implement complex DHS changes, as well as their commitment for improved health care quality and responsiveness to broader developmental needs.

REFERENCES

African National Congress. (1994). *The Reconstruction and Development Programme: A policy framework.* Johannesburg, SA: Umanyano Publications.

Auditor-General of South Africa (AGSA). (2011). *Consolidated general report on provincial audit outcomes 2010–11.* Pretoria, SA: AGSA.

Barron, P., & Asia, B. (2001). The district health system. In A. Ntuli, F. Suleman, P. Barron, & D. McCoy (Eds.), *South African health review 2001* (pp. 17–48). Durban, SA: Health Systems Trust.

Blecher, M., Kollipara, A., de Jager, P., & Zulu, N. (2011). Health financing. In A. Padarath & R. English (Eds.), *South African health review 2011* (pp. 29–48). Durban, SA: Health Systems Trust.

Bossert, T. (1998). Analyzing the decentralization of health systems in developing countries: decision space, innovation and performance. *Social Science & Medicine, 47*(10), 1513–27. https://doi.org/10.1016/S0277-9536(98)00234-2

Buhlungu, S., & Atkinson, D. (2007). Politics: Introduction. In S. Buhlungu, J. Daniel, R. Southall, & J. Lutchman (Eds.), *State of the nation: South Africa 2007* (pp. 27–34). Cape Town, SA: Human Sciences Research Council.

Cameron, R. (2006). Local government boundary reorganisation. In U. Pillay, R. Tomlinson, & J. du Toit (Eds.), *Democracy and delivery: Urban policy in South Africa* (pp. 76–106). Cape Town, SA: Human Sciences Research Council.

Coovadia, H., Jewkes, R., Barron, P., Sanders, D., & McIntyre, D. (2009). The health and health system of South Africa: Historical roots of current public health challenges. *Lancet, 374* (9692), 817–34. https://doi.org/10.1016/S0140 -6736(09)60951-X

Council for Medical Schemes. (2011). *Annual report 2010/11.* Pretoria, SA: Council for Medical Schemes.

Day, C., Barron, P., Monticelli, F., & Sello, E.T. (2009). *The District Health Barometer 2007/2008.* Durban, SA: Health Systems Trust.

Department of Health. (1995). *The implementation of a district health system: Obstacles to overcome and issues to resolve.* Pretoria, SA: Department of Health.

Department of Health. (1997). *White paper for the transformation of the health system in South Africa. Government Gazette,* no. 17910. Pretoria, SA: Department of Health.

Department of Health. (2010). *National Department of Health strategic plan 2010/11– 2012/13.* Pretoria, SA: Department of Health.

Department of Health. (2011). *National health insurance in South Africa: Policy paper.* Government Notice: 657 of 12 August 2011, Government Gazette, no. 34523. Pretoria, SA: Department of Health.

Department of Health. (2012). *Annual performance plan of the National Department of Health strategic – 2012/13.* Pretoria, SA: Department of Health.

Department of Health. (2015). *National health insurance for South Africa: Towards universal health coverage – Version 40.* Pretoria, SA: Department of Health.

Department of Health & Health Policy Coordinating Unit. (1995). *A policy for the development of a district health system for South Africa.* Pretoria, SA: Department of Health.

Development Bank of South Africa. (2008). *Health sector roadmap.* Johannesburg, SA: DBSA.

Gilson, L., Morar, R., Pillay, Y., Rispel, L., Shaw, V., Tollman, S., & Woodward, C. (1996). *Decentralisation and health system change in South Africa.* Johannesburg, SA: Health Policy Coordinating Unit.

Harrison, S., & Qose, M. (1998). Health legislation. In A. Ntuli (Ed.), *South African health review 1998* (pp. 17–28). Durban, SA: Health Systems Trust.

HST. (2002). *South African health review.* Durban, SA: Health Systems Trust.

HST. (2008). *District management study, a national summary report: A review of structures, competencies and training interventions to strengthen district management in the national health system in South Africa.* Durban, SA: HST.

Integrated Support Teams. (2009). *Review of health over-spending and macro-assessment of the public health system in South Africa: Consolidated report.* Pretoria, SA: ISTs.

Matsoso, M.P., & Fryatt, R. (2013). National health insurance: The first 18 months. In A. Padarath & R. English (Eds.), *South African health review 2012/13* (pp. 21–36). Durban, SA: Health Systems Trust.

McCoy, D. (1996). *Free health care for pregnant women and children in South Africa: An impact assessment.* Durban, SA: Health Systems Trust.

McIntyre, D.E., & Doherty, J.E. (2009). Health care financing and expenditure: Progress since 1994 and remaining challenges. In H.C.J. Van Rensburg (Ed.), *Health and health care in South Africa* (pp. 377–411). Pretoria, SA: Van Schaik.

Naledi, T., Barron, P., & Schneider, H. (2011). Primary health care in SA since 1994 and implications of the new vision for PHC re-engineering. In A. Padarath & R. English (Eds.), *South African health review 2011* (pp. 17–28). Durban, SA: Health Systems Trust.

National Planning Commission. (2011). *National development plan: Vision 2030.* Pretoria, SA: National Planning Commission.

National Treasury. (2012a). *Budget review 2012.* Pretoria, SA: National Treasury of the Republic of South Africa.

National Treasury. (2012b). *Financial status of provincial departments under administration: Presentation to the portfolio committee on public service and administration, 6 June 2012.* Cape Town, SA: Parliament.

National Treasury. (2013). *Budget review 2013.* Pretoria, SA: National Treasury of the Republic of South Africa.

National Treasury. (2015). *Intergovernmental fiscal review 2015 – Provincial budgets and expenditure review 2010/11–2016/17.* Pretoria, SA: National Treasury of the Republic of South Africa. http://www.treasury.gov.za/publications/igfr/2015/prov/default.aspx

Public Service Commission. (2011). *Fact sheet on the duration of employment per grade of senior management service members.* Pretoria, SA: PSC.

Republic of South Africa. (1996). Constitution of the Republic of South Africa 1996, Act 108 of 1996. http://www.gov.za

Republic of South Africa. (1999). Public Finance Management Act, no 1 of 1999. Pretoria, SA: Government Printer.

Republic of South Africa. (2000). Municipal Structures Amendment Act of 2000. Pretoria, SA: Government Printer.

Republic of South Africa. (2004). National Health Act no 61 of 2003. Government Gazette, no. 469 (26595), 1–94.

Rispel, L. (2016). Analysing the progress and fault lines of health sector transformation in South Africa. In A. Padarath, J. King, E.-L. Mackie, & J. Casciola (Eds.), *South African health review 2016* (pp. 17–23). Durban, SA: Health Systems Trust. http://www.hst.org.za/publications/south-african-health-review-2016

Rispel, L.C., de Jager, P., & Fonn, S. (2016). Exploring corruption in the South African health sector. *Health Policy and Planning*, 31(2), 239–249. https://doi.org/10.1093/heapol/czv047

Rispel, L., & Moorman, J. (2010). Analysing health legislation and policy in South Africa: Context, process and progress. In S. Fonn & A. Padarath (Eds.), *South African health review 2010* (pp. 127–44). Durban, SA: Health Systems Trust.

Rispel, L., & Moorman, J. (2013). Health sector reforms and policy implementation in South Africa: A paradox? In J. Daniel, P. Naidoo, D. Pillay, & R. Southall (Eds.), *New South African review 3: The second phase – tragedy or farce?* (pp. 239–60). Johannesburg, SA: Wits University Press.

Rispel, L., & Setswe, G. (2007). Stewardship: Protecting the public's health. In S. Harrison, R. Bhana, & A. Ntuli (Eds.), *South African health review 2007* (pp. 3–17). Durban, SA: Health Systems Trust.

Statistics South Africa. (2017). *2017 mid-year population estimates: Statistical release P0302*. Pretoria, SA: Statistics South Africa.

Van Rensburg, H.C.J. (Ed.). (2004). *Health and health care in South Africa*. Pretoria, SA: Van Schaik.

Van Rensburg, H.C.J., & Pelser, A.J. (2004). The transformation of the South African health system. In H.C.J. Van Rensburg (Ed.), *Health and health care in South Africa* (pp. 109–70). Pretoria, SA: Van Schaik.

van Ryneveld, P. (2006). The development of policy on the financing of municipalities. In U. Pillay, R. Tomlinson, & J. du Toit (Eds.), *Democracy and delivery: Urban policy in South Africa* (pp. 157–84). Cape Town, SA: Human Sciences Research Council.

WHO. (1978). *Alma-Ata 1978: Primary health care*. Geneva, Switzerland: World Health Organization.

Chapter Seven

Brazil: Local Government Role in Health Care

MARTA ARRETCHE AND ELIZE MASSARD DA FONSECA

Introduction

This chapter presents the main characteristics of the Brazilian decentralized system of health care, known as the Unified Health System (Sistema Único de Saúde, SUS). It analyses the main traits of a system that has been built since the early 1990s, as a result of the 1988 Federal Constitution. SUS is a nationwide, publicly funded health care system, which citizens are entitled to access on a free and universal basis. It is called unified because the decentralized provision of health care is made under the ultimate authority of the federal health ministry.

As we demonstrate in this chapter, the Brazilian health system can be described as a devolved model of decentralization, since health provision is attributed to subnational units, mainly municipalities, with the financial support of both the federal government (which contributes the largest share of revenues) and states. In this model, subnational governments have a narrow to moderate space to make decisions about delegated health policies. Although subnational units are free to adhere or not to the Brazilian health system, the structural features of the Brazilian federation and the way services are vertically organized, along with federal-led nationwide rules, make adhesion to the Unified Health System a dominant strategy for subnational governments.

Structural Features of the Federation

The current configuration of the Brazilian public health care was framed by the 1988 Federal Constitution (1988 FC) when the Unified Health System was approved. Since its very inception, it was conceived as a three-tier system of responsibility in which health care provision should be shared by the Union, states, and municipalities. Indeed, the creation of the current Brazilian health system involved three structural changes in health policy as compared to the previous model. The first embeds citizens' right to health care. The 1988 Constitution replaced the previous insurance-based model, which was restricted to workers in the formal labour market, with a free, universal, and publicly funded model.

Second, the previous centralized system – in which all providers were hired by a bureaucratic federal agency – was replaced by a decentralized one. Article 198 of the 1988 FC states that health responsibilities should be shared by the three government tiers. Moreover, Article 30, Section VII states that municipalities should have constitutional responsibility for health care provision, with states and the federal government providing technical and funding support. As a result, municipalities play a key role in health care provision in Brazil.

Third, a previous bureaucratic decision-making model, entirely managed by federal agencies located in the Brasilia Federal District, was replaced by one in which health councils at all three government levels were established to participate in health decisions (Article 198). There are two very important modes of participation: 1) civil society participation through thousands of local and state-level health councils; and 2) municipal and state-level representatives' participation in health decisions as well as federal-state-municipal health commissions.

Complementary laws – particularly the National Health Law (NHL) – framed decentralization in such a way that municipalities are meant to have the competence to plan and organize local health actions along with managing and executing primary health care provision. Article 18 (items I and II) of the NHL also charges municipalities with responsibilities for planning, programming, and organizing service provision with state governments. The federal government retained financing and coordination responsibilities.

Despite the intent of such legislation to grant major responsibility to municipalities, the Union came to be the most important arena for decision-making on health care policy as a result of a number of decisions in the process of establishing the Brazilian health system beginning in the early 1990s. Local governments as well as most states are heavily dependent on federal-driven rules. Transfer rules were framed in such a way as to bind federal revenue flows towards subnational governments – either states or municipalities – in their implementation of federal-set programs. If states or municipalities do not comply with federal-driven rules, then they are not entitled to receive federal transfers earmarked for health.

The notion that the unified system is also a hierarchical one, under the authority of the federal Ministry of Health, has meant that in practice local municipalities, the main providers of health care services, are far from having full autonomy to make decisions about health policies, in spite of their constitutional status as fully recognized members of the federation. In practice, however, municipal policies are directly influenced by the national government since, unlike other federations, Brazilian municipalities are not under the direct authority of the states.

In fact, one of us has shown (Arretche, 2013) that policy decision-making in Brazil cannot be fully understood if we assume it is an extreme case of demos-*constraining* federalism whose institutions were expected to systematically defeat initiatives to provide national goods (Samuels & Mainwaring, 2004; Stepan, 2004). Instead, Brazil could be better described as displaying demos-*enabling* elements, since political institutions enable the federal government to deal with national problems without infringing on the rights of subunits, since these are framed to limit the possibilities of minority groups blocking the will of the majority. The 1988 Federal Constitution empowers the federal government to initiate legislation in all policy areas, including those with decentralized implementation, so that in most policy areas constitutional amendments are not needed for approving legislation. Legislation on the finances, policies, and spending of subnational units can be submitted to Congress either as complementary laws – addressed to regulate the Constitution – or ordinary laws. Thus, many policy changes affecting subnational affairs can be approved in Congress by a simple plurality of votes.

Nevertheless, this *demos-enabling* elements in policy decision-making does not imply that states do not play an important role in health care provision. In fact, states are responsible for providing technical support for municipalities, and in many cases states are responsible for specialized hospitals and clinics, since most Brazilian municipalities cannot afford to fund them. In the event that state governors decide to implement policies aimed at giving support to municipalities, this support can make a significant difference in the health outputs of such municipalities (Arretche, 2000). In sum, both states and municipalities provide health services under a nationwide framework whose standards and rules are set by the national government.

Funding

Articles 195 and 198 of the 1988 FC state that the Union, states, and municipalities are all responsible for funding the health system. Figure 7.1 clearly shows that the Union contributes the most for the health system funding, even though this participation has been declining since the adoption of decentralization. The Union contributed to roughly 75 per cent of health funding from 1980 until the early 1990s, when decentralization – particularly towards municipalities – was introduced.

Figure 7.1 Public-sector health spending by government level, Brazil, 1980–2008

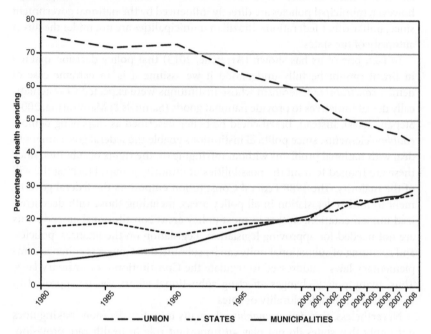

Source: CONASS (2011)

Since then, the Union's share of total public-sector spending on health has steadily declined, down to 43.5 per cent in 2008. At the same time, both the municipalities' own revenue and the states' financing increased to 27 per cent by 2008.

Nevertheless, despite the growing importance of subnational participation on health care funding, the Union remains the level of government which spends the most on public health, mainly through its transfers to states and municipalities, since all expenditures on health care are made through subnational governments. As federal transfers are the most important source of municipalities' revenue in Brazil, as we shall see, the increasing participation of municipalities in health care funding means that the Union was successful in binding municipalities' revenues – either self-generated ones or upper-level transfers – to local health spending.

As a universal system which is free at the point of service, all public-sector health spending is financed by general taxes and the contributions to the social security system. These are earning related and collected only from workers in the formal job market, although benefits are distributed according to the pay-as-you-go model and all citizens above 65 years old are entitled to at least one minimum-wage payment.[1]

The funding of public health has been a highly controversial issue in Brazilian politics, though. On the one hand, the adoption of a public, universal, and free health provision system largely augmented the number of beneficiaries. Until 1988, when entitlement to public health care was insurance based, only workers in the formal job market as well as autonomous insurance-payers were enrolled in the public health care. In the late 1980s, formal workers made up 40 per cent of the total population in Brazil (Curi & Menezes-Filho, 2006). Free and universal access, by its turn, enlarged beneficiaries to the entire population, a change that has exerted strong spending pressure.

The 1988 Constitution framers meant to fund universal health care by both general taxes and social security contributions. However, in 1993 the Ministry of Social Security stopped making transfers to the Ministry of Health in order to manage its own social security deficit. To compensate for this revenue loss, the Ministry of Health got approval to create a specific federal tax addressed to fund health care. The tax – the Provisory Contribution on Banking Accounts (Contribuição sobre a Movimentação Financeira, CPMF) – was implemented in 1994 but became so unpopular that it was eventually abolished in January 2008. Two factors contributed to its demise. First, and most important, it was levied on each check of bank account holders, making it highly visible each time an account holder paid a bill. Second, CPMF was not earmarked exclusively to health care. Framed in such a way, it became the target of a tax revolt led mainly by middle-class organizations, whose representatives blamed CPMF for taking money away from taxpayers without giving anything back. After its abolition, subsequent initiatives to launch a federal tax similar to CPMF faced strong opposition and could not garner enough support to get approved.

It is important to note that the public sector is not the only provider of health services in Brazil. Private insurance has provided health care to nearly one-quarter of the Brazilian population. In 2012, 47 million inhabitants (26.3 per cent of the population), mainly employees in large and medium-size enterprises as well as middle-class families, were enrolled in private insurance schemes (ANS, 2012). This share is slightly higher than that found in 1998, when

---

1 Brazilian citizens are entitled to one minimum-wage retirement benefit regardless of previous contributions to the social security system, provided that they are 65 years old and poor (that is, living in households whose per capita earnings are below one-quarter of the minimum wage).

24.5 per cent of the Brazilian population was enrolled in private schemes (Bahia et al., 2006, p. 956), and a bit higher than the 22 per cent figure estimated for 1990 (Bahia, 2001). Hence, the private provision of health care insurance seems to have slightly increased the last twenty years. This inference should be taken with some caution though, because data for the late 1980s and early 1990s is based on estimations.

Private spending was estimated to be around 56.4 per cent of the total spending on health in 2009, 57.2 per cent of which was out-of-pocket, 41 per cent from private health insurance, and almost none of which was from international sources or donors (World Health Organization, 2012). Coverage by private insurance depends on the type of plan hired, although minimum standards are controlled by the National Health Agency (Agência Nacional de Saúde or ANS). Drugs and medicines are not covered by private insurance though, and the public system only provides a limited number of them for free.

Organization of the Public Health Care System

Since its very inception in 1988, the governance, financing, and administration of the Brazilian health system was conceived as unified and hierarchical, where high-level direction comes from the Union but mainly operational decisions on service delivery were decentralized to the states and municipalities. Moreover, civil society participation was also conceived as a central pillar of the new institutional arrangement, with compulsory health councils at all three government levels. Finally, subnational government participation in policy decision-making was institutionalized in the early 1990s by means of intergovernmental deliberation committees.

Figure 7.2 presents the organization of the public-sector health system in Brazil. By constitutional mandate, the Ministry of Health is responsible for financing, coordinating the provision of services, collecting data, and evaluating outcomes and performance. The Ministry of Health is also entitled to set the legal frameworks and policies that subnational governments are in charge of implementing.

As a result of pressure by state and municipal health authorities, a three-tier government commission (Comissão Intergestores Tripartite, CIT) was created in July 1991. The CIT is composed of an equal number of representatives (fifteen members) of the Ministry of Health, the Council of State-Level Health Authorities (Conselho Nacional de Secretários Estaduais de Saúde, CONASS), and the Council of Municipal-Level Health Authorities (Conselho Nacional de Secretários Municipais de Saúde, CONASEMS). The CIT is meant to be a forum where three-tier managers of health policies negotiate how policies will be implemented.

Figure 7.2 Sistema Único de Saúde (SUS) organizational structure

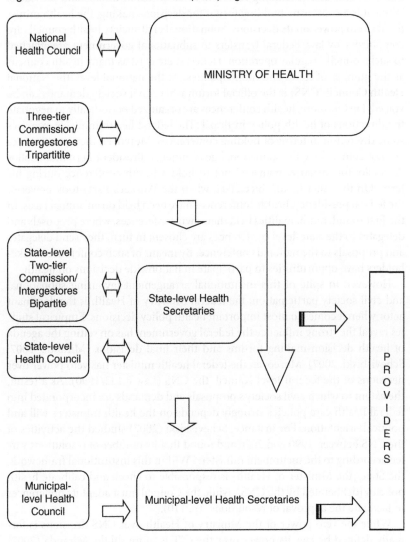

Civil society has a say on policymaking at the national level by means of the National Health Council (created in 1990), which is composed of representatives of a large spectrum of stakeholders, including the insurance industry, business, and users including representatives of health unions and providers. While it is a consensus-building forum for decision-making, the health minister has veto power on its decisions. Subnational civil society health councils are compulsory by law. Federal transfers to subnational government are attached to such councils' regular operation. Hence, there exist as many health councils as the number of states and municipalities. At the national level, the National Health Council (CNS) is the official forum where civil society demands can be voiced. Furthermore, health conferences are organized periodically to negotiate the directions of health policy in Brazil. The federal health ministry exercises some discretion in terms of holding conferences. Moreover, these conferences are not compulsory for subnational governments. President Fernando Collor de Mello, for instance, managed not to hold a health conference during his term. On the other hand, since 2004, when the Worker's Party took power of the federal presidency, health conferences have been held on an annual basis. In the first round, municipalities held their own conferences, where proposals and delegates to the state-level conferences are chosen; in turn, they send delegates and proposals to the national conference. By means of such conferences, stakeholders have opportunities to participate in nationwide decisions on health.

However, in spite of this institutional arrangement favouring subnational and civil society participation, the federal Ministry of Health is the dominant actor when it comes to most important health policy decisions. Empirical studies reveal the strong influence the federal government has on setting the agenda of health decision-making forums and their final decisions (Miranda, 2007; Schevisbiski, 2007). Moreover, the federal health minister has veto power over decisions of the federal-level council, the CNS (Law 8.142/1990). As a result, the extent to which civil society's proposals and demands are incorporated into federal health care policies strongly depends on the health minister's will and political orientation. For instance, Schevisbiski (2007) studied the activities of the CNS between 1990 and 2006 and found that its number of resolutions varied according to the incumbent minister: "Within this institutional framework, the State [the Minister of Health] is responsible to check and calibrate health policies [deliberated by the CNS], while the Council must adapt its preferences to facilitate the approval of resolutions" (p. 110).

While the veto power of the Ministry of Health over CNS decisions is formally defined by law, its power over the CIT is more subtle. Miranda (2007) analysed CIT's normative documents from 2001 to 2002 and interviewed governmental actors. She found evidence of asymmetrical power among CIT's members favouring the federal level. The Ministry of Health's agenda is prioritized (despite the disagreement of other members), and ad hoc norms and institutional requirements are unilaterally set by the federal ministry without submission to intergovernmental negotiation. Nevertheless, interviewees agreed that CIT plays an important role in the decentralization process by allowing a permanent space of negotiation between the three levels of government. It also improved their capacity to perform health programs and actions, by negotiating the role of each level on policy implementation.

Since 1993, the health ministry's earmarked transfers to states and municipalities have become automatic. This means that they are distributed according to legally and publicly known rules so that subnational governments are entitled to receive them as long as they comply with federal rules. Transfers are usually broken up into several different programs so that subnational governments have to accomplish the requirements of each program in order to receive the total amount of health care transfers to which they are legally entitled.

Since President Fernando Henrique Cardoso's government (1995–2003), there has been an impressive increase in the Ministry of Health's capacity to evaluate and audit subnational systems. Consequently, the ministry has had detailed oversight on the state and municipal health care programs' performance.

States and municipalities are required to have segregated health funds – that is, health funds are separated from other budget items. Transfers from the federal government to states and municipalities as well as from states to their own municipalities are made on the basis of "health fund to health fund." Each state and municipality has its own health account where transfers are directly allocated. This way of organizing health transfers is meant to insulate them from local disputes over revenues transferred from the federal government.

States and municipalities are also expected to have their own civil society health councils. Indeed, federal law stipulates that transfers should not be made in the absence of an active health council. Subnational health councils are required to supervise health spending. Hence, in cases where the state or municipal health council does not approve the "health budget," transfers are automatically suspended until the accountability process is concluded. Empirical studies also show that effective civil society participation in health councils is highly dependent on the commitment of health authorities. If elected and appointed officials are not in favour of civil society participation, they often have means to make councils less influential (Cortes, 2002; Labra, 2002).

At the state level, state health secretaries negotiate the provision of services with municipal health secretariats. The state-level two-tier commission is the main forum where such negotiations take place. Region-wide strategies for service provision are the main subject of such meetings.

Both municipalities and states are allowed to contract private providers. Municipalities can qualify themselves to be responsible for more specialized health care services. In such cases, they directly contract and pay private hospitals and clinics. Otherwise, they remain responsible only for the direct provision of primary health care. When this is the case, the state government becomes responsible for specialized services.

As a result, the health ministry does not make direct payment to private providers. Private providers have an important role in more specialized health services provision. In 2013, private providers were solely 1.4 per cent of the 50,096 basic health units, whereas the private sector represented 33 per cent of the 9,867 hospitals, 95 per cent of the 160,488 specialist outpatient clinics, 68 per cent of the 6,711 polyclinics, and 92 per cent of the 19,460 diagnostic and therapy centres (authors' calculations based on data of the National Survey of Health Facilities, Cadastro Nacional de Estabelecimentos de Saúde).[2]

In other words, units for primary health care are mainly owned and managed by municipalities, whereas secondary and tertiary provision is mainly in the hands of private providers, which sell services to either municipal or state governments.

Health System Decentralization

A key issue on the comparative study of decentralization refers to the decision space of subnational governments. Table 7.1 summarizes data on the extension of choices attributed to subnational governments in different health functions – namely finance, service organization, human resources, access rules, and governance rules – based on Bossert's (1998) decision space approach.

Finance

Municipalities are responsible for primary care health provision, while states play an important role in the supply of specialized services, particularly hospitals. In fact, large and medium-size cities are in charge of hiring private hospitals and managing public ones, whereas state governments have the responsibility of hospital service supply in many medium and small cities. Hence, stating that there is a kind of division of labour between states and municipalities according to which municipalities are in charge of primary care and states manage secondary care somehow oversimplifies the actual arrangements. However, such

---

2 DATASUS, Cadastro Nacional de Estabelecimentos de Saúde. http://cnes.datasus.gov.br (retrieved 10 October 2013).

Table 7.1 Local decision space at the subnational level, Brazil

Function	Indicator	Range of Choice		
		Narrow	Moderate	Wide
Financing				
Sources of revenue	Intergovernmental transfers as % of total subnational health spending	Varies for municipalities but generally dependent on federal funds	Varies for states but half of states depend on federal funds for at least 50% of their spending	
Allocation of expenditures	% of total local spending is explicitly earmarked by higher authorities		12% for states 15% for municipalities	
Fees contracts	Range of prices local authorities are allowed to choose	No choice or narrow range		
Contracts	Number of models allowed	Contracts regulated by Law 8666 (federally regulated)		
Service organization and delivery				
Hospital autonomy	Range of autonomy for hospitals		Contracts regulated by CA 19/98	
Insurance plans	Choice of how to design insurance plans	No insurance plans are allowed for the public sector		N/A
Payment mechanisms	Choice of how providers will be paid (incentives and non-salaried)	Contracts regulated by CA 19/98		
Required programs	Specificity of norms for local programs	Ruled by Ministry of Health's decrees		

(Continued)

Table 7.1 Local decision space at the subnational level, Brazil (Continued)

Function	Indicator	Range of Choice		
		Narrow	Moderate	Wide
Human resources				
Salaries	Choice of salary range		Ceiling by (federal) Fiscal Responsibility Law	
Contracts	Contracting non-permanent staff	Defined by the Constitution		
Civil service	Hiring and firing permanent staff	Defined by the Constitution		
Access rules				
Targeting	Defining priority population	Defined by higher authority		
Governance rules				
Facility boards	Size and composition of boards			Defined by subnational governments
District offices	Size and composition of local offices			Defined by subnational governments
Community participation	Size, number, composition, and role of community participation		Defined by federal law	

simplification is useful for the following analysis, which is based on the average pattern in Brazil.

Figure 7.3 illustrates Brazilian states' and municipalities' revenue sources and decentralized health funding. Due to the great variation in taxing and revenue capacities of Brazilian states and municipalities, Figure 7.3 uses a series of box plots. Given this variation, measures like "average" or "median" do not fully display the Brazilian context. Data refers to the average of three fiscal years (in 2008–10) in order to avoid biases associated with measuring only one discrete point in time. Box plots are calculated for all Brazilian states and municipalities.

The first box plot (on the extreme left of Figure 7.3) shows the own-taxation capacity of Brazilian municipalities. It presents the share of self-generated taxes on a municipality's total budget. The fact that the black line, within the box (the median value), is around 5 per cent means that 50 per cent of Brazilian municipalities get at most 5 per cent of their total budget through own-source revenues. Hence, one-half of Brazilian municipalities display very low capacity to generate revenues based on the taxes they are entitled to levy. Stars represent outliers, meaning that few municipalities get more than 15 per cent of their total budget by means of their own tax collection. This box plot shows how unequal Brazilian municipalities are when it comes to obtaining self-generated revenue.[3]

Low self-generating revenue capacity should not be interpreted as a consequence of municipalities' fiscal laziness, or their desire to pass the financial responsibility to higher levels of government; rather, it is the result of the narrow space for taxation municipalities face because of the federal legislation.[4]

As a result, most Brazilian municipalities are heavily dependent on state and federal transfers, their most important source of revenue. If Brazilian municipalities were to rely only upon own-source taxation, their average budget would be US$76 per capita in 2010. Federal and state transfers increased municipal average annual per capita revenues to US$657 in 2010. Moreover (and very

---

3 This outcome is the result of a combination of the nationwide taxation rules and a constitution that limits the tax-raising powers of local governments. Municipalities are only authorized to tax urban real estate, services, and property transfers. In addition to limiting the types of taxes municipalities can levy, the rules for fixing the rates for each type are set by the national legislature.

4 If, for example, the citizens of a given municipality agreed to pay a dedicated tax to fund their own health services, they would be forbidden to do so by the Federal Constitution. Moreover, wealth is highly concentrated in some municipalities, and the majority are not affluent enough to get sufficient revenues to fund adequate health services, even should they expend considerable efforts in tax collection.

important for guaranteeing free political competition at the local level), such transfers lie outside political bargaining, since the rules for their distribution are constitutionally mandated.

The most important federal transfer is called the Municipality Participation Fund (MPF) and is based on a share of 23.5 per cent of the total collection of two exclusive federal taxes: income tax and the tax on industrialized products. Ten per cent of this amount is earmarked for division among the state capitals, with each individual quota calculated by a formula directly related to population and inversely related to the state's per capita income. The remaining 90 per cent is divided as per a formula that favours less populous municipalities.[5]

Constitutional transfers (federal and state) have only been moderately effective in reducing revenue inequality between Brazilian municipalities for at least three main reasons. First of all, cross-municipality revenue-raising capacities are highly unequal, as illustrated in Figure 7.3. Arretche (2011) calculated the Gini coefficient for Brazilian municipalities' self-generated tax receipts and found values around 0.50, with 1 being most unequal and 0 being most equal. Second, states' constitutional transfers are distributed according to the amount collected in each town. Hence, their entry into municipalities budgets reduces the Gini coefficient to 0.45. It is left up to the federal MPF to reduce revenue inequality, and there is in fact a sharp reduction in inequality when this revenue source is added to local own-source revenues. All Brazilian municipalities considered, the Gini coefficient for self-generated plus MPF falls to around 0.30. MPF's allocation rules are based on an understanding that the smaller the city, the poorer it is. As a result, the rules favour the smallest municipalities instead of the neediest ones.

Besides constitutional transfers, municipalities are entitled to get upper-level transfers earmarked to health care, both from the federal and state governments. Entitlement to federal earmarked health transfers is universal in the sense that both municipalities and states receive them as long as they fullfil federal requirements. Such transfers are usually labeled as voluntary, in the sense that the national government is not bound by the Constitution to distribute them. However, their allocation rules are so institutionally embedded in SUS operations that they are no longer considered voluntary.

The second box plot in Figure 7.3 presents data on the importance of federal earmarked health transfers to municipalities in terms of the share of such transfers in the average total budget of Brazilian municipalities. For 50 per cent of Brazilian municipalities, federal earmarked health transfers represent more

---

5 A number of other transfers from the federal government to local ones are also constitutionally based. For a detailed account, see Afonso and Araújo (2006).

Figure 7.3 States' and municipalities' revenue sources, Brazil, 2008–10

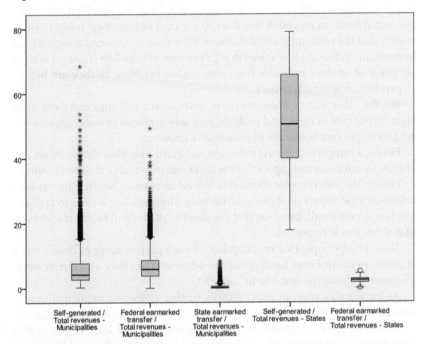

Source: National Treasury

than 10 per cent of their total budget. Stars represent outliers – those municipalities for which federal earmarked health transfers represent more than 20
per cent of their total budget. Hence, these health transfers represent a similar
share of municipalities' total budgets as their own-source revenues.

The third box plot shows Brazilian states' earmarked health transfers to their
own municipalities. The black line in this box plot is close to zero. It means that,
as a general pattern, states' earmarked health transfers to their own municipalities have a minor role in funding the latter's health policies. Once more, stars
represent outliers, where state-government contributions to municipalities
exceed 10 per cent of their total budget. It means that only for a small number of Brazilian municipalities does the state-level contribution represent some
meaningful share of the total budget of those municipalities. The conclusion is
straightforward: federal earmarked health transfers are far more important for
a municipality's budget than state ones.

The fourth box plot shows states' self-generated revenue capacity. The black line here is around 50 per cent. It means that for half the Brazilian states self-generated taxation represent less than 50 per cent of their total budget, which means that the remaining amount comes from federal transfers. Moreover, the vertical line below the box shows that 25 per cent of Brazilian states get at most 40 per cent of their revenues from own-source taxation, so they are heavily dependent on federal transfers.

For the other half of Brazilian states, own-source revenues represent more than 50 per cent of their total budgets, and only a quarter of states get between 65 and 80 per cent by means of own-source taxation.

Hence, a comparison between the first and fourth box plots clearly shows that the own-source revenue capacity of the states outstrips that of the municipalities.

Finally, the fifth box plot shows that federal earmarked health transfers have relatively little impact on states' total budgets. The black line is close to zero and the box is very small, meaning that the share of the federal health transfers on states' budgets is minuscule.

These results imply that municipalities have a narrow range of choice when it comes to control over fiscal resources, whereas states have a moderate range of choice (refer to the first line in Table 7.1).

As for the allocation of expenditures, neither states nor municipalities are entirely free to make their own decisions. Constitutional Amendment 29 (CA 29), approved in 2000, establishes that states should spend at least 12 per cent of their revenues on health care, while municipalities' threshold should be 15 per cent. The earmarking of the Union's revenues to health were not defined until December 2011, when a law stipulated that the federal government's annual spending on health should be calculated on the basis of the amount spent in the previous year, with an increase based on a two-year rolling average of gross national product (GNP).

However, the spending of states and municipalities have exceeded this formula. Therefore, their decision space in terms of health spending is moderate in practice even if narrow in theory. Moreover, state governors and municipal mayors have the discretion to decide where they are going to spend within the health envelope; for example, they can decide to spend either in poorer or more affluent cities and neighbourhoods.

As for the use of income from fees, the decision-making space is *narrow* since neither municipalities nor states are able to charge any fees. As for contracting private providers, the subnational decision space is narrow, since rules are set by the federal legislation. For instance, the law (Lei 8666/1993) mandates the establishment of competitive bidding procedures for public procurements of goods and services. All ministries and subnational governments are required to publish bid notices open to all participants wishing to take part in a price quotation procedure.

Service Organization

Primary care is provided only by municipal governments, which means that basic services are mainly public. Specialized health services though can be provided by private hospitals and clinics by means of contracts with either states or municipalities. Hospital contracting is at the core of a lively debate that divides the health policy community as well as political parties. Some support contracting out as the best way to achieve efficiency, while others fiercely resist incorporating what they call private logic into the public health care system.

States and municipalities can directly contract either private or public specialized health care providers. However, their autonomy to set the rules of such contracts is limited by federal laws. Article 22 of the Brazilian Federal Constitution says that the Union has exclusive authority to set the general rules as regards subnational budget elaboration and public contracts. Moreover, contracting out by subnational governments is regulated by the 19/1998 and the 29/2012 constitutional amendments, which set (i) rules for contracting out; (ii) thresholds on subnational health spending; and (iii) which spending items can be taken as health expenditures. As a result, we classified subnational governments as having a moderate space to decide about either hospital autonomy or provider payment.

To protect the free and universal nature of the Brazilian health system, the federal government does not allow states and municipalities to permit or regulate private health insurance. Private insurance plans are regulated by an independent agency, the National Health Agency (ANS). Hence, subnational governments have narrow decision space – indeed, no space – on health insurance.

Basic Operational Norms (NOBs) enacted by the Ministry of Health are the main instrument for the federal coordination of decentralized programs. Programs launched by the Ministry of Health are accompanied by transfers in such a way as to make it attractive for subnational governments to adhere to them. Moreover, as shown earlier, the limited tax-raising capacity of most municipalities makes it very attractive for them to adhere to federal-led programs in order to enlarge their budgets. As a result, the Ministry of Health uses its spending power to get subnational compliance with federal programs.

Given their political autonomy, subnational governments have the constitutional authority not to adhere to federal-led programs. Although non-adherence is indeed a formal option, there is a price to be paid for non-compliance: no money from the Ministry of Health. Subunits are also entitled to launch their own programs, provided they fund them with their own resources. For example, until 2012, the 26 states and the Federal District along with 4,589 (out of 5,564) municipalities adhered to the Pact for Health, launched in 2006 by the Ministry of Health, and signed a document which defined the health responsibilities and goals of state and local governments. Subnational compliance with federal norms is based on a free calculation of their costs and benefits. In practice, given that the overwhelming majority of subunits need federal transfers for implementing health care, compliance is the dominant strategy. Hence, we classified the range of choice in required programs as *moderate*.

Human Resources

There are no limits on the salaries to be paid for subnational governments' health workers as long as no more than 60 per cent of the budget is spent on personnel, a ceiling set by the federal Fiscal Responsibility Law. Since states and municipalities are allowed to pay whatever they deem appropriate or necessary within this overall cap, the decision space of subunits regarding salaries is moderate.

However, rules for either non-permanent staff contracts or permanent civil servant contracts are defined by the federal law. In fact, Article 27 of the 1988 FC gives the Union exclusive authority to set the rules on the general norms for all types of contracts to be made by the three levels of government and their companies. As a result, amendments to the Constitution had to be presented before Congress in order to make it possible for subnational governments to hire non-permanent and permanent staff. This was particularly relevant for hiring semi-skilled health workers in charge of community-based health care. Hence, constitutional amendments 34/2001 and 51/2006 were also approved to allow, respectively, for health professionals to have cumulative contracts with states and municipalities, and for the states to hire agents responsible for community-wide health services. Hence, the decision space for staff contracts is moderate, since general guidelines for contracting health staff are set by federal rules and subnational governments have little discretion regarding the contract rules. Although constitutional amendments managed to overcome obstacles to contract health staff, such rules are still under the exclusive authority of the Union.

Access Rules

Subnational governments have no autonomy at all to define the target beneficiaries of health policy. The Brazilian Constitution says that access to health care should be public, free, and universal. Hence, the decision space for states and municipalities is classified as narrow.

Governance Rules

Subnational governments have a wide decision space when it comes to the size and composition of facility boards, as well as district offices. However, community participation is compulsory. Having a local or state-level health council entitled to supervise health programs and the health fund's accounts is a condition to receive federal transfers.

General rules about the composition of health councils are also set by federal laws. The Ministry of Health's legal provision sets the minimum number of users, providers, and governmental representatives each subnational council must have. However, it is up to mayors and governors to set the rules and procedures through which civil society representatives will be elected. Moreover, they are entitled to define which organizations will be taken as representatives of civil society. As a result, mayors and governors have some room to manipulate the composition of councils (Arretche, 2004). Moreover, empirical evidences show that advocacy groups organized in NGOs have many more seats than social movements in health councils (Perez, 2010). Hence, we classified the range of choice regarding community participation as moderate.

Capacities of Subunits

Measuring the capacities of subunits to accomplish their health tasks must take into account the division of responsibilities between the three levels of government. As already said (refer to Figure 7.1), the federal government does not have health provision responsibilities in Brazil. Instead, only states and municipalities are in charge of providing health care. Moreover, only municipalities are in charge of basic health care services. Hence, we cannot employ the same indicator to compare the state capacities of different government levels, since the type of professionals required for the central government to perform its own tasks is not the same as those required by the subunits.

The per capita number of public-sector health employees – either permanent or non-permanent staff – might be a candidate for comparison. However, even such an indicator would be controversial since different tasks to be accomplished imply different measures of efficiency to the ratio of employees/population. As a result, comparisons would be of little analytical value.

Finally, it does not make sense to analyse municipalities and states as if they were homogeneous. Instead, inequality among states and among municipalities is a central characteristic of Brazilian subunits; thus any average value for states and municipalities would be of little analytical value. Such methodological issues might explain why there are no systematic and comprehensive studies on the health managerial capacity of subnational units in Brazil. Yet evidence presented thus far – particularly on the revenue side – allow us to say that there is likely to be wide variation among them in this regard.

As a result, we opted for the per capita number of physicians and health workers as a very rough indicator of the capacity of municipalities to perform their health competences. Since the Brazilian health system is integrated to the extent that states and municipalities do not compete with one another regarding the provision of services, it does not matter whether a health professional is employed by a municipality or state government. As a result, Figures 7.4 and 7.5 show the capacity of the Brazilian health system to provide health services in a decentralized way.

Both maps show there is a sharp difference between subunits when it comes to their health capacities. The spatial distribution of per capita physicians is highly unequal. Physicians are concentrated in the wealthiest regions in the south while there are physician shortages in the poorer northern regions.[6]

Inequality is less pronounced when it comes to health workers, though. Figure 7.5 shows that, although subunits' capacity is far from equal, since some municipalities have less than two health professionals per 1,000 inhabitants and others have more than six, the spatial distribution of health professionals does not seem to be so much associated with spatial inequality of economic activity as physician distribution is.

While this spatial distribution of health capacities is counterbalanced to some extent by federal transfers, these transfers are insufficient to equalize revenue capacity among subunits. In the absence of federal transfers, subunits' spending capacity would be even more unequal than they end up being.

Recent Health Policy Changes and Trends

Brazilian public health care is conceived as a three-tier system of responsibility which aims to be a free, universal, and publicly funded one. Its current configuration is the result of a twenty-year building process

---

6 The Ministry of Health is considering importing physicians to fulfil positions in the northern regions of Brazil. Such a proposal has proved to be a highly controversial issue though. See the article on Valor Economico, on 14 May 2013: "Governo descarta validação automática de médicos estrangeiros," http://www.valor.com.br/brasil/3123146/governo-descarta-validacao-automatica-de-medicos-estrangeiros.

Figure 7.4 Per capita number of physicians by municipality, Brazil, 2012

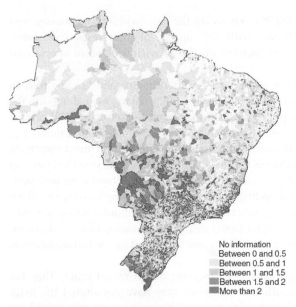

No information
Between 0 and 0.5
Between 0.5 and 1
Between 1 and 1.5
Between 1.5 and 2
More than 2

Source: DATASUS, Cadastro Nacional de Estabelecimentos de Saúde. Available at http://cnes.
datasus.gov.br. Retrieved 10 August 2012.

Figure 7.5 Per capita number of health workers by municipality, Brazil, 2012

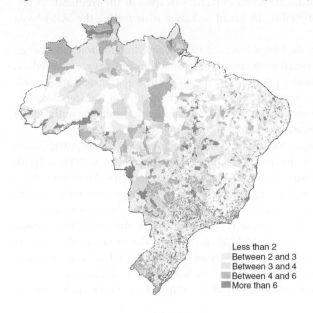

Less than 2
Between 2 and 3
Between 3 and 4
Between 4 and 6
More than 6

Source: DATASUS, Cadastro Nacional de Estabelecimentos de Saúde. Available at http://cnes.
datasus.gov.br. Retrieved 10 August 2012.

culminating in municipalities receiving the responsibility to manage and deliver primary health care with the support of their respective states, whose responsibilities are focused on the provision of more specialized and hospital services.

The federal government performs a key coordinating and funding role. In the Brazilian case, decentralization of health policymaking went along with the centralization of health policy decision-making in the sense that subnational units have a narrow to moderate space to make decisions about a number of key dimensions of health policy. In practice, the Union is the most important arena for decision-making on nationwide health care policy, with states and municipalities heavily dependent on federal transfers to fund their own policies. Indeed, the Union spending power implies that compliance with federal rules is the dominant strategy for transfer-dependent subunits. As a result, subnational health providers are far from having full autonomy to make decisions about health policies, in spite of their constitutional status as full members of the federation.

Health policy changes have been incremental in recent years. They fall short of full-fledged health reforms, since they have not altered the main pillars of the Brazilian health system. The SUS paradigmatic principles have been respected by different presidents regardless of their party affiliation. In fact, introduced changes aimed more at handling the challenge of providing adequate health care to all citizens – in spite of the tremendous territorial inequality prevailing in Brazil – than at dismantling the SUS's basic foundations.

First of all, the way the Union has exercised its coordination role does not go unchallenged. Subnational units complain of what they call an excessive federal intrusion into their health programs by means of the way transfers are framed. So they ask for more flexibility, since the fragmentation of transfers into different programs accompanied by detailed requirements limits the authority of states and municipalities to decide their own policies.

From 2004 to 2006, negotiations on this issue took place in the participation forums, particularly in the three-tier commission. As a result, in 2006, a health ministry's decree replaced the more than a hundred earmarked transfers with a model in which transfers are aggregated according to health functions, namely primary care, secondary and tertiary care, preventive care, pharmaceutical assistance, and SUS management (Portaria 399/2006 and 699/2006). Hence, under President Luiz Inácio Lula da Silva, transfer rules towards subunits were changed. Such changes remain strongly attached to federal-led programs and projects though, meaning that the Brazilian health system remains one in which the federal government holds the power to set the rules nationwide. In sum, the historically narrow to moderate decision space for subnational governments persisted despite these changes in the transfer system.

Second, handling the challenge of providing equal access to health care along with the efficient supply of services has driven many changes in the way services are organized. Out of the 5,565 Brazilian municipalities, 2,515 have less than 10,000 inhabitants. Small and poor municipalities face great challenges in providing medium- and high-complexity health services, a challenge that ranges from attracting physicians to installing the necessary infrastructure and facilities. To address this problem, presidential decree 7508/2011 created 419 health regions, based on the current distribution of health facilities, clustering neighbouring municipalities. These health regions should be managed by municipal health secretariats. It aims at creating the conditions for municipalities to share more complex service facilities. For such a purpose, a contract must be signed. The Public Action Organizing Contract (Contrato Organizativo da Ação Pública da Saúde, COAP) sets the authorities and obligations of the three government levels referring to the integration and organization of region-wide health services, including funding obligations. The state government is responsible for coordinating the implementation of these contracts, and the Ministry of Health is responsible for coordinating the content, execution, and evaluation of these contracts.

One key provision of Decree 7508 is its emphasis on cooperation for health planning, which should include measurable goals and monitoring strategies. Instruments such as the state-level and municipal health plans, the Annual Health Programming (detailing actions and services, annual goals, evaluating indicators, and corresponding health budgets), the General Programming of Health Actions and Services (an agreement between government levels about region-wide quantitative outputs and resources), and, finally, the Management Report (listing of accomplishments) were introduced. As a whole, such instruments aim at providing for improved region-wide collaboration between government levels to gain efficiency on more complex health service provision. Once more, such changes did not alter any of the traditional pillars of SUS, although they meant to address its most outstanding shortcomings.

ACKNOWLEDGMENTS

The authors thank Sergio Piola, André Bonifácio, Patrícia Ribeiro, Luiza Guimarães, Nilson do Rosário Costa, and Edgard Fusaro.

REFERENCES

Afonso, J.R.R., & Araújo, E.A. (2006). Local government organization and finance: Brazil. In A. Shah (Ed.), *Local governance in developing countries* (pp. 381–417). Washington, DC: World Bank.

ANS. (2012). Beneficiários de planos privados de saúde, por cobertura assistencial (Brasil – 2003–2012). http://www.ans.gov.br/perfil-do-setor/dados-gerais. Retrieved 31 August 2012.

Arretche, M. (2000). *Estado federativo e políticas sociais: Determinantes da descentralização*. Rio de Janeiro, Brazil: Revan.

Arretche, M. (2004). Toward a unified and more equitable system: Health reform in Brazil. In R.R. Kaufman & J.M. Nelson (Eds.), *Crucial needs, weak incentives* (pp. 155–88). Washington, DC: Woodrow Wilson Center/Johns Hopkins University Press.

Arretche, M. (2011). Federalism and territorial equality: A contradiction in terms? *Dados, 5*, 587–620.

Arretche, M. (2013). Demos-constraining or demos-enabling federalism? Political institutions and policy change in Brazil. *Journal of Politics in Latin America, 5*(2), 133–50.

Bahia, L. (2001). Planos privados de saúde: Luzes e sombras no debate setorial dos anos 90. *Ciência & Saúde Coletiva, 6*(2), 329–39. https://doi.org/10.1590/S1413 -81232001000200005

Bahia, L., Raggio Luiz, R., Salm, C., Leal Costa, A.J., Kale, P.L., & Cavalcanti, M. de L.T. (2006). O mercado de planos e seguros de saúde no Brasil: Uma abordagem exploratória sobre a estratificação das demandas segundo a PNAD 2003. *Ciência & Saúde Coletiva, 11*, 951–66.

Bossert, T.J. (1998). Analyzing the decentralization of health systems in developing countries: Decision space, innovation, and performance. *Social Science & Medicine, 47*(10), 1513–27.

CONASS. (2011). *Sistema Único de Saúde: Coleção Para Entender a Gstão do SUS*. Vol. 1. Brazil: Conselho Nacional de Secretários de Saúde (CONASS).

Cortes, S.M.V. (2002). Construindo a possibilidade da participação dos usuários: Conselhos e conferências no Sistema Único de Saúde. *Sociologias, 7*, 18–49.

Curi, A., & Menezes-Filho, N.A. (2006). O mercado de trabalho brasileiro é segmentado? Alterações no perfil da informalidade e nos diferenciais de salários nas décadas de 1980 e 1990. *Estudos Econômicos, 36*(4), 867–99.

Labra, M. (2002). *A qualidade da representação dos usuários nos conselhos distritais de saúde no Rio de Janeiro e a dimensão associativa (Relatório de pesquisa)*. Rio de Janeiro, Brazil: ENSP/Fiocruz.

Miranda, A. (2007). Intergovernmental health policy decisions in Brazil: Cooperation strategies for political mediation. *Health Policy and Planning, 22*(3), 186–92. https://doi.org/10.1093/heapol/czm004

Perez, O. (2010). *A representação em arenas extraparlamentares: Os conselhos gestores de políticas públicas* (unpublished doctoral dissertation). University of São Paulo, São Paulo, Brazil.

Schevisbiski, R.S. (2007). *Regras institucionais e processo decisório de políticas públicas: Uma análise sobre o conselho Nacional de Saúde (1990–2006)* (unpublished master's thesis). University of São Paulo, São Paulo, Brazil.

Samuels, D., & Mainwaring, S. (2004). Strong federalism, constraints on the central government, and economic reform in Brazil. In E.L. Gibson (Ed.), *Federalism and democracy in Latin America* (pp. 85–129). Baltimore, MD: Johns Hopkins University Press.

Stepan, A. (2004). Toward a new comparative politics of federalism, multinationalism, and democracy: Beyond Rikerian federalism. In E.L. Gibson (Ed.), *Federalism and democracy in Latin America* (pp. 29–84). Baltimore, MD: Johns Hopkins University Press.

World Health Organization. (2012). *World health statistics 2012*. Geneva, Switzerland: World Health Organization.

Chapter Eight

Decentralization of Health Policy and Services in Mexico

MIGUEL A. GONZÁLEZ BLOCK, LUCERO CAHUANA HURTADO,
LETICIA AVILA-BURGOS, AND EMANUEL OROZCO

Structural Features of Mexico

The United States of Mexico is a federal republic of thirty-one autonomous states and the Federal District of Mexico City, seat of the federal government. Mexico has 114 million inhabitants, of whom 10 million live in the Federal District and over 20 million in its metropolitan area. Mexico is classified as an upper-middle-income country, with a purchasing power parity GDP per capita of $15,000 in 2010, ranked 78th in the world (World Bank, 2011). Yet Mexico is also a country with regionally contrasting wealth and health disparities across north and south: GDP per capita in 2010 was as high as US$26,285 in states like Nuevo Leon and as low as US$6,356 in Chiapas. Infant mortality rates vary across these two states, from 10.0 per 1,000 live births to 19.5, respectively.

The Mexican Constitution creates three orders of government – federal, state, and municipal – with formal autonomy to elect authorities and to levy taxes. Health functions are assigned by the Constitution to the three orders of government. The federation has the capacity to issue guidelines and execute actions in matters of national importance, such as health regulation and disease control and prevention. States are responsible for health service provision within their jurisdictions, complemented by federal actions that go beyond their borders. However, the federation also has the capacity to provide health services directly within state jurisdictions, chiefly to comply with its constitutional obligations relating to social security for private and federal employees. Mexican federalism is symmetric according to Requejo (2010), with all states sharing an equal relationship and no special groups being recognized. However, constitutional amendments have given indigenous groups greater recognition and a modest capacity for self-government.

In comparison to other federations, the Mexican has a low degree of constitutional decentralization.

Mexico is a developing democracy, with alternation of government parties since 2000. Its political regime, however, still bears the influence of the authoritarian corporatist state, dominated by the Partido Revolucionario Institucional (PRI), established after the Mexican Revolution ended in 1917. Corporatism can be defined as a peak hierarchical organization of different groups (e.g., peasants or unionized workers) to negotiate and accommodate their collective interests. It has also been an effective means of elite control of these economic groups. Patronage is a key mechanism of assuring loyalty, whereby leaders are co-opted within various state organs such as Congress and official trade unions. Corporatism has meant that the federal government retains a large degree of central power – mostly vested in the control of fiscal resources and of massive service organizations. The federal government exerts influence on state governments in the health arena through earmarked resource transfers, coordination agreements, and mixed federal-state service provider organizations. While a greater share of federal resources is now being spent at the state level, it remains unclear whether this has resulted in state governments achieving more power and authority.

This chapter first outlines the development of the Mexican health system from the perspective of federal-state relationships. The chapter then focuses on the decentralization triggered by one major health reform implemented in the last ten years – the policy of universalizing financial protection known as Seguro Popular. This policy was formulated by the first government led by an opposition party that replaced the PRI-dominated government in 2000. Seguro Popular introduced an innovative, demand-based financing mechanism for the non-insured. Transfers from the federation to state health providers increased throughout the decade, significantly closing the financing gap between the insured and the non-insured.

States were also given incentives to increase their own investments, and significantly greater amounts of resources were administered even within tighter constrains, thereby leading state actors to become more prominent. These changes gave greater bargaining power to the states and thus were clear trends in favour of decentralization. Yet the continued segmentation of the health system and the still centralized control of social security agencies have limited health system decision-making by the states. Furthermore, fiscal resources have remained highly controlled at the federal level overall, constraining the capacity of states to engage more meaningfully in resource pooling and allocation – the hallmark of a truly decentralized regime.

The Foundation of the Mexican Health System

The Mexican Constitution of 1917 mandates the federation to ensure the stability of employer-labour relationships and gives employers a clear responsibility for occupational health and well-being. The Constitution further mandates the federation to ensure the public health of the nation through what is today the Ministry of Health. A General Board of Health gives the president executive power to address epidemic threats. Provisions are made in Article 4 of the Constitution for the federal and state governments to address "general health," understood as health responsibilities not allocated in Article 123 of the Constitution to the realm of labour relationships and thus to social security institutions. Given the corporatist authoritarian regime that predominated throughout the twentieth century, the federal government dictated health policy and implemented it either through highly centralized institutions under Article 123 or through arrangements involving state governments in various degrees.

The current health system was influenced by economic policies to establish a protectionist industrialization regime during World War II. This led in 1943 to the upgrading of the Department of Health into a full-fledged Ministry of Health and Assistance, charged with providing medical care to the peasantry and the urban poor. Simultaneously, the government implemented the constitutional mandate for an obligatory social security system through the Social Security Law and the Mexican Institute of Social Security (Instituto Mexicano del Seguro Social or IMSS). IMSS was established with very wide powers, charged with directly collecting contributions from employers, employees, and the federal government; investing those funds in proprietary medical infrastructure; and directly operating the infrastructure for the exclusive benefit and use of employees. A bipartite contributory scheme was also established for the most powerful groups of organized peasants. Federal bureaucrats, as well as members of the army and navy, kept their own health and pension schemes, following a constitutionally mandated separation of labour regimes. In 1959, the diverse pension and medical insurance schemes of federal bureaucrats were merged in the Institute for Social and Security Services for State Workers (Instituto de Servicios y Seguridad Social de los Trabajadores del Estado or ISSSTE).

IMSS and ISSSTE governance is through delegated bodies of the federal government, administered by a presidentially appointed director and a technical committee of stakeholder representatives. Social security institutes are deconcentrated at state and substate levels, and professional, clerical, and janitorial workers are organized under their respective trade unions, today affiliating over 500,000 workers. Social security institutes have undergone a slow process of managerial reform through deconcentration, particularly for budgeting and purchases. Relationships with the Ministry of Health and with state health systems remain scant, with federal social security directors being invited to attend State Health Boards meetings as a means of supporting health system coordinating, mostly for public health campaigns.

Compulsory insurance and national governmental control of IMSS and ISSSTE have played a key role in fuelling industrial growth and bolstering the government's power through resolving the multiple health-related disputes that had characterized industrial relations prior to the institution of the national schemes (Brachet-Márquez, 2010; González-Block, Leyva, Zapata, Loewe, & Alagón, 1989). Indeed, industrial and government workers' participation is organized at delegation levels through trade union appointees, excluding the representation of non-unionized affiliates.

IMSS, ISSSTE, and the Secretaría de Salud (SSA) were set to grow following demographic and industrial trends during the economic boom of the 1950s and 1960s. However, in the 1970s, a slowdown of the economic model became evident with the accumulation of the urban and rural poor. The highly centralized and segmented health system was perceived as a threat by an emerging critical voice of intellectuals and political parties and by government itself. The diagnostic included massive, out-of-control federal expenditures (especially within development and public health programs), redundant infrastructure, and ineffective protection for the poor. Federal policymakers were also concerned with the segmentation of health institutions and the inefficiency of investments to extend health coverage under the paradigm of primary health care. The federal government responded, mandating IMSS in 1973 to fund and manage a medical care program for the rural poor through a separate and minimally endowed infrastructure. This program has survived and is now called IMSS Prospera, although today funding is allocated fully through fiscal resources of the national budget.

Decentralization and Federalization of the National Health System: 1983–2000

The government of Miguel de la Madrid (1982–8) faced the impending social crisis through social development programs in close coordination with state governments and across sectors. The administration developed a vision of a decentralized national health system under the stewardship of the Ministry of Health, with greater separation of functions between regulators and providers and especially with stronger state ministries of health, envisioning them as fully capable of autonomous health service provision through state-appointed ministers of health mobilizing both federal and state funding

(Soberón et al., 1983). The Mexican Constitution was reformed to enshrine the Right to Health Protection – more specifically, the right to gain access to health services. No changes were made, however, to the employer obligations to provide social security for their employees, thus justifying the continued autonomy of IMSS and other social security institutes such as ISSSTE and state-level agencies for local bureaucrats.

The government initiated the policy of decentralization through the reform of the General Health Law (Ley General de Salud), enabling the devolution of local health and operational responsibilities to state governments, even while the federal government remained responsible for financing and coordinating health sectors and regulating safety and risk protection. Each state was offered generic legislation adapted to local circumstances through state health laws, thus ensuring intergovernmental coordination through a more formal procedure than the administrative agreements of the past. Table 8.1 is the decision space map, describing decentralization outcomes in terms of the degree of choice achieved in the period between 1983 and 2012.

In spite of the constitutional and legal change, the concept of a decentralized national health system failed to be legislated in the General Health Law, being mentioned only in passing as a generic coordination mechanism. This left the federal Ministry of Health with limited legal capacity to address social security inequality and inefficiency (Ibarra et al., 2013). Nonetheless, the Constitutional Right to Health gave ideological impetus to the Ministry of Health in two broad directions: 1) to claim greater resources as a federal health sector regulator and thus to become more credible vis-à-vis powerful stakeholders in IMSS and ISSSTE; and 2) to decentralize vertical public health programs and medical services for the non-insured to the state governments under a primary health care approach, thus overcoming resistance by program stakeholders and trade unions. Furthermore, a new General Health Board convened state health ministers on a quarterly basis to consult them on critical policy developments and to monitor policy implementation.

Based on the legal and institutional reforms, the federation signed decentralization agreements with the states, stipulating public health and stewardship responsibilities for the entire population as well as service provision for the non-insured (Arredondo, 2003). These agreements were signed in two waves. The first was in the mid-1980s with twelve state governments that went on to integrate all services for the non-insured, including the IMSS special service for the extreme poor. The second wave of decentralization was in the mid-1990s with the remaining twenty states, once SSA gave up on the effort to integrate the IMSS-operated special program. IMSS had shown vigorous opposition to losing this program from the start of decentralization, arguing that

Table 8.1 Provincial health department decision space in Mexico (hospital and primary health care services)

Function	Indicator	Range of Choice		
		Narrow	Moderate	Wide
Financing				
Sources of revenue	Intergovernmental transfers as % of state health spending	Most funding by federal government		
Allocation of expenditures	% of state spending that is explicitly earmarked by national health authorities	Per capita transfers tied to affiliation to Seguro Popular. Most allocated to interventions in federal catalogue or public health programs		
Income from fees and contracts	Extent to which state governments can raise funds through user fees for hospital services		User fee levels set by states but charged only for hospital care outside federal catalogue of interventions	
Service organization and delivery				
Hospital autonomy	Range of autonomy for hospitals		Diverse forms of autonomy possible but little used	
Payment mechanisms	Choice of how providers (hospitals and PHC facilities) paid (incentives and non-salaried)		Incentives can be freely designed and paid but little used	
Physician autonomy	Choice of how physicians are governed, organized, and paid	Governance through trade union rules or temporary consulting contracts		
Required programs	Specificity of norms for provincial programs	Highly regulated federal public health programs		

(Continued)

Table 8.1 Provincial health department decision space in Mexico (hospital and primary health care services) (Continued)

Function	Indicator	Range of Choice		
		Narrow	Moderate	Wide
Human resources				
Salaries	Choice of salary range	Set by federal government through negotiations with national trade unions		
Contracting	Contracting non-permanent staff		Freedom to contract through diverse formulas and salaries but pressures to trade-unionize	
Civil service	Hiring and firing of permanent staff	Restricted by national trade unions		
Access rules				
Targeting	Defining priority populations	States restricted to care for informal-sector workers, self-employed, and part of the poor		
Governance rules				
State health administration	National rules limiting size, number, or composition of state health department		States can determine ministerial structures and degree of state government decentralization, but most follow a set pattern	
District offices	Size and composition of local offices		Follow federal program needs and funding	
Facility (hospital) boards	Size and composition of boards	Most hospitals are centralized state government bodies and have no boards		
Community participation	Size, number, composition, and role of community participation	States can designate community-based bodies to monitor a narrow range of federally prescribed quality indicators		

state governments were dismantling it. Indeed, this program had given IMSS the capacity to demonstrate a modicum of redistribution, if only through an administrative role, thus defending its privileged funding in the face of economic crisis and stagnation (Avila-Burgos, Cahuana-Hurtado, Pérez-Núñez, Aracena-Genao, & Hernández-Peña, n.d.; González-Block, 1996; González-Block et al., 1989).

The results of the first wave of decentralization were considerable, though limited. Responsibility for federal health infrastructure up to secondary-level hospitals was transferred to state decentralized corporations (Organismo Público Descentralizado or OPD). State ministers of health or directors of health services were given administrative power to hire and fire federal personnel, although the national trade union maintained its strong negotiation and worker protection powers. While decentralization did not fully integrate state and federal hiring policies, working conditions and pay scales across states were integrated. Payment of wages for federal employees was deconcentrated to the states. New posts strengthened tactical roles for the management of key programs. However, this was done mostly through federal posts, and no efforts were made to stimulate richer states to fill them. Between 1983 and 1995, posts more than doubled, from 65,133 to 140,939 (Nigenda & Ruiz, 1999). In this context, the federation retained all powers to accredit professionals, define job profiles, set wages, and hire personnel, including the power to negotiate directly with the trade union on bylaws, training, incentives, and occupational health and safety. As already stated, state authorities were given only limited powers to solve human resources conflicts. Given this very narrow decision space, ineffective negotiations in the context of a strong national union have led to important urban-rural imbalances.

On the financing front, decentralization led the federation to assign block grants to states (Arredondo, Parada, Orozco, & García, 2004; Avila-Burgos et al., n.d.). However, states' high degree of dependency on federal resources meant little real autonomy in practice (Avila-Burgos et al., n.d.; Moreno, 2001). The economic crisis also meant important budgetary constraints (González-Block, Tapia-Conyer, & Olaiz, 1994). Federal and state block grants and other resources were managed through a single provider established in each of the thirty-two states as a deconcentrated (OPD) entity of the state governments. OPDs are governed by a board chaired by the state minister of health and with the participation of one representative of the federal Ministry of Health, one trade union representative, and two representatives of various state government bodies. Although OPDs are governed by state laws and are therefore independent of the federal government, the participation of federal representatives overseeing the federal majority funding gives OPDs a mixed state-federal character.

The OPD board meets every two months for administrative oversight and troubleshooting. In most states, the OPD director is also the state's minister of health and the OPD operates as the ministry of health. The director-minister post is usually funded by the federation through the OPD role, although in some cases it is a state post. In other states the ministry of health has a small structure of its own and is fully funded by state governments. Yet in these cases, there is a very close functional relationship, with the OPD director responding directly to the minister in day-to-day business and the latter serving as chair of the OPD board.

Social development policy was transformed during the PRI administration (1988–94) with its vision of social liberalism. Health decentralization came to be perceived as a cumbersome and conflict-ridden way of responding to the challenges of poverty and social development. Instead, a strengthened Ministry of Health implemented vertical programs such as universal immunizations, in part through World Bank funding, to achieve universal coverage of twelve essential interventions as part of the anti-poverty program. The fight against poverty was mounted through a federally controlled cash-transfer program known as Solidarity. The administration that came to power in 1994 implemented a new program, the Education and Health Program (PROGRESA), with the innovation of transparent beneficiary identification and cash allocation on the basis of families performing according to the rules.

The conditional cash-transfer program, now called Prospera, today benefits 5.8 million families living in extreme poverty. This program is operated along highly efficient and transparent procedures. State health providers were given the minor role of monitoring attendance to primary health care clinics and reporting to federal authorities in charge of affiliation and payment.

The rift in the health sector between decentralized (with devolution agreements integrating all public health infrastructure for the non-insured) and deconcentrated states (no agreements and maintenance of SSA and IMSS Prospera infrastructure) was resolved when the remaining states signed agreements and newly appointed ministers of health joined the National Health Board. However, IMSS Prospera was not integrated; instead it was protected as a mechanism to deliver federal aid without state government intrusion. The new structure enabled the federation to improve the delivery of vertical programs, particularly immunizations and the Health Service Coverage Extension Program (PAC), which channelled World Bank funding to twelve essential interventions accompanying the fight against poverty.

During the 1988–94 administration, the responsibilities of state ministries of health were streamlined to support the federally funded goals (Arredondo et al., 2004) through a new program of deconcentration within states, implemented through a project to develop MOH jurisdictions to strengthen Local Health Systems (Sistemas Locales de Salud, SILOS). SILOS aimed to increase the technical capacity of personnel at the local level (jurisdictions) of the state ministries of health, as well as to give them greater autonomy for planning, budgeting, and managerial decision-making (González-Block, 1996).

SILOS should have led to a widening of the states' decision space, given that federal funds could have been more freely allocated by local authorities to attain federal goals and objectives. However, deconcentration within states failed from a lack of coordination between federal, state, and jurisdictional financing regulations; resources thus remained earmarked according to historical trends. Analysis of the program's evaluation results suggests that, contrary to expectations, strengthening the capacity of local officers was negatively associated with primary health care performance. This may have been due to an unrecognized targeting of the worst-off jurisdictions for capacity strengthening followed by a lag between training and performance improvements that were not captured through the evaluation. Indeed, this negative association not only eventually disappeared but was more significantly positive in the jurisdictions that managed to attain greater autonomy (González-Block, 1996). These results suggest the potential that local autonomy had to make the best use of capacity strengthening efforts towards improved performance.

The PRI federal administration of 1994–2000 introduced a vision of a strengthened federal pact, "federalization," formulated through a reform to the Law of Fiscal Coordination establishing Resource Transfer Funds to States (FASSA). FASSA specified budgeting and programming criteria for personal health services and for public health, including an innovative resource-allocation formula using state indicators, among them medical infrastructure, health personnel, federal taxation, contributions to social security, and mortality and poverty. Funds were earmarked for use by the OPD in exchange for the provision of a basic package of health services that was agreed by the federation and the states through the General Health Board. The main purpose of FASSA was to increase the decision space of state ministries of health so that they would have greater capacity to budget in line with locally identified health needs. However, earmarking also gave the federation control over funds that had to be transferred to state treasuries (Diario Oficial de la Federación, 1996; Gobierno de la República Mexicana, 1999; Moreno, 2001).

The FASSA reform had important consequences for state governments (see Figure 8.1 for the current financial architecture). Initially, states became responsible for the direct execution of 25 per cent of total health expenditure in 1994 (González-Block & Brown, 1997), but this figure nearly trebled to 70 per cent by 1999. Furthermore, this expenditure was only reported to the state congress, while the Ministry of Health was informed only of general health outcomes (Moreno, 2001). A clearer separation of functions was thus established between the federation as the principal and the state executives as agents, accountable to the federal Ministry of Health and to the state congresses (Moreno, 2001; Noriega, Huitrón, & Matamoros, 2006).

While federal resources increased, FASSA failed to stimulate state health expenditure, with the exception of state capital expenditures. Indeed, state contributions were mostly directed to investments through earmarking by the state government (Arredondo & Orozco, 2006; Arredondo et al., 2004; Noriega et al., 2006). In spite of the resource-allocation formula, FASSA led to greater inequity of financial allocations across states given its failure to override the inertia of historical funding following the existing infrastructure. An important exception was the subsidy by PROGRESA-Oportunidades to primary health care clinics in rural areas, although this did not substantially shift funding equity because of the low levels of funding involved (Arredondo & Orozco, 2006; Arredondo et al., 2004; Noriega et al., 2006).

The political climate in which federalism was nurtured also promoted a new vision of separation of provision, financing, and stewardship functions, espoused by researchers and the policymaking elite within the federal Ministry of Health (Frenk, Lozano, & González Block, 1994). This vision aimed less to support decentralization or privatization per se than to strengthen the federal government's capacity to make wise investments in the health sector and to deliver more value.

The failure of decentralization and other federal policies since the 1980s to bring about greater participation of state authorities, and especially to empower them to override the financial imbalances and the inequity of health service provision for the non-insured, was seized upon in 2000 when the new administration of Vicente Fox came to power.

National Health System Integration and Social Protection in Health: 2000–12

President Vicente Fox, the first president supported by a political party that was not the PRI, espoused a vision of strengthening democracy and equity. As his minister of health he selected Julio Frenk, who complemented this vision by highlighting the importance of a more equitable health system to attain the long-cherished Right to Health as well as to sustain economic development. He focused on the importance of financial protection for health and on universal access to prepaid, comprehensive health services.

Health financing was seen as the core of the problem, given historically low levels of investment, imbalance between federal and state contributions

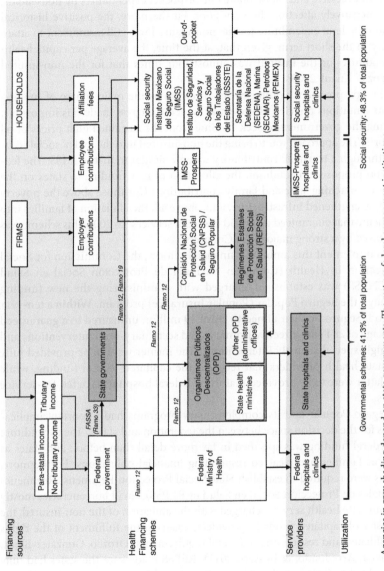

Figure 8.1 Financial flows to public federal and state health service providers in Mexico, 2012

Agencies in grey shading depend on state governments. The rest are federal government institutions.
Modified from Gómez-Dantés et al. (2011) and Avila-Burgos et al. (2016).
Note: Coverage rates based on Romero-Martínez et al. (2013).

and across states, high expenditure on human resources, historical financing of states following the inertia of infrastructure, and, chief among all, the high levels of excessive and catastrophic out-of-pocket expenditures by households, most negatively affecting the very poor. Furthermore, the positive historical trend in federal expenditure for the non-insured was still insufficient to attain equity in the short term, given that, at the time, the average per capita health expenditure for the insured was almost four times that for the non-insured (Arzoz & Knaul, 2003).

The Fox presidency proposed fiscal reform as the main source of funding for its ambitious policies. However, a divided Congress made this impossible, forcing the government to seek funding from the sustained high prices of oil exports. The approach was to bring the non-insured into the fold of social security through a tripartite contributory scheme similar to that of IMSS. The federation proposed to condition the allocation of new funding to states on the basis of matching state and family contributions (for those above the poverty line), strengthened infrastructure, and, above all, the affiliation of families into a scheme that guaranteed a prepaid basket of services. In 2002, this scheme was approved by a strong majority in Congress.

To implement this ambitious financial reform, the Commission for Social Protection in Health (Comisión Nacional de Protección Social en Salud or CNPSS) was established, charged with administering the new funding through the Seguro Popular (Popular Insurance) program. Within a ten-year period, Seguro Popular aimed to enrol 49 million uninsured to a guaranteed package of 284 cost-effective primary- and secondary-level interventions and 45 high-specialty, costly interventions. The former were to be provided fully by state health providers that received the capitated federal funding, while the latter were to be provided mainly by federal hospitals on a fee-for-service basis.

Seguro Popular and its complementary programs had important implications for the decision space between the federation and states. The expenditure of federal funding was specified in far more detail than before, and states as well as families had clear corresponding financial obligations. Furthermore, states were required to establish State Social Protection Regimens (Regímenes Estatales de Protección Social en Salud or REPSS), small bureaucracies mostly within state health services charged with the affiliation of the non-insured, the transfer of capitated funds to providers, ensuring the fulfilment of the rights of affiliates, and responding to federal requirements (Orozco, González-Block, Rouvier, Arredondo, & Bossert, 2011). REPSS made sure the states had fully accredited facilities capable of providing the package of interventions. Funds were used chiefly to bolster health human resources, maintain infrastructure, and purchase medicines; federal funds could not be used for investments or to hire administrative personnel.

As Table 8.1 shows, decentralization had narrow and medium outcomes, basically because this process couldn't involve social security and private institutions. The financing function had the greatest challenge given that the federal government continued to be the predominant funder. More prominent – although still moderate – were the outcomes achieved for the human resources and health services organization functions, since state governments did take up important responsibilities. The 2003 reform introduced relevant changes to financing and governance, although no substantial changes were made to the federal government's predominant role, nor did they imply expanding the degree of choice in other functions.

The Mexican government's health system is currently characterized by two relatively autonomous sets of institutions (Figure 8.1). The first set includes federal and state funds and service provider organizations serving the population excluded from social security schemes, including the Ministry of Health; state health services; CNPSS; and the IMSS Prospera program (although this last is operated by a social security institution). Today, 41 per cent of the population is formally covered by these institutions and services. The second set of institutions includes the social security agencies serving private- and government-sector workers (predominantly IMSS for private-sector workers); the Institute for Social Security and Services for Civil Servants (ISSSTE); and various agencies for military, the oil industry, banking, and state and municipal services. As a whole, the social security agencies formally cover 48.3 per cent of total population (Avila-Burgos et al., 2016).

The following subsections analyse the changes brought about by Seguro Popular on federal-state relationships with respect to financing, governance, access rules, human resources, and health service organization.

Financing

Financing of health services between the federal government and the states has shifted since 2000, mostly from changes brought about by Seguro Popular. Proportionately more funding by the federation implies greater centralization, given its greater control of decision spaces through financing accountability. Similarly, proportionately higher contributions by state governments should translate into greater decentralization. However, it is important to note the effect of specific financial control mechanisms over federal or state control and, therefore, the implications of greater central control of funding.

Seguro Popular funding by the federation was allocated from "Ramo 12" (Figure 8.1), an expenditure line earmarked by Congress for administrative expenditures of the Ministry of Health. This gave the federal Ministry of Health greater control over resources, as they had to be transferred to OPDs based on yearly agreements tied to specific performance benchmarks. Ramo 12 funds were in part allocated on the basis of a set of criteria designed to ensure equity across states, as well as to compensate for increased funding and improved performance by states.

The state governments were required to provide the State Solidary Contribution directly to state health providers using sources of their own choosing, although most have used their line items for investment in infrastructure. Families also contribute a share; however, families with incomes below the fourth decile of income were exempted. Although both states and families join the scheme on a voluntary manner, no state has failed so far to sign or renew the annual agreements, chiefly because of the funding incentives (López-Arellano & Blanco Gil, 2008).

Seguro Popular meant an 11.9 per cent financial increase to Mexico's total health expenditure, going from US$891 PPP to US$916 PPP per capita between 2001 and 2010 or 0.8 per cent of GDP, from 5.4 per cent in 2001 to 6.2 per cent in 2010.[1] However, public-sector health expenditure did not shift significantly, as it was 45 per cent of the total health spending in 2001 and had only reached 47.3 per cent by 2010. Furthermore, family contributions for Seguro Popular were not as expected, with only 7.2 per cent of the expected 54 per cent of affiliated families contributing (Nigenda et al., 2010). This shortfall can be explained by a lax affiliation process that enabled higher-income families to be classified in a lower category, itself the result of the high incentive by the state and federal authorities to affiliate without regard to the low level of financing that would be attained through family contributions. State authorities thus demonstrated the capacity to interpret federal rules according to their own interests while still being consistent with those of the federation.

Seguro Popular meant greater resources for state health authorities, but states were somewhat limited in their ability to make allocation decisions since they had to account for all expenditures according to line items. The federal government stipulated strict maximums and minimums for expenditures: maximums of 40 per cent for human resources and 30 per cent for medicines, and minimums of 20 per cent for public health programs and 5 per cent for

---

1 Purchasing Power Parity (PPP): These are currencies or price deflators used to convert different currencies to a common one. The conversion process seeks to equalize purchasing power between countries, eliminating differences in price levels. http://www.inegi.org.mx/est /contenidos/Proyectos/INP/PPC/Presentacion.aspx.

infrastructure maintenance. Furthermore, REPSS are formally free to contract other public or private providers, but they are under strong pressure to finance state health services.

Evidence from the operation of Seguro Popular in four states with contrasting socio-economic conditions indicates that, in spite of the line-item ceilings and limitations to spend outside of state-controlled services, REPSS and state health authorities do have a degree of choice on how resources are allocated (Orozco et al., 2011). States are in general able to allocate funding to public or private providers using diverse payment formulas such as line-item in-kind or in-cash subsidies, capitation, and case-based payment, although the latter two are mostly used for private providers. REPSS are also able to purchase medicines from a diverse range of providers and through different purchasing mechanisms, widening their decision space. With increased federal and state funds, state health authorities experimented with what can be termed a systemic centralization, where they managed more federal resources but also took a greater number of strategic decisions to adapt them to local needs and to allocate state funding.

Importantly, CNPSS kept the allocation of a separate Catastrophic Expenditure Fund for high-specialty services, amounting to 18 per cent of the total expenditure on health, fully under federal control. This fund has been made available to private providers, including to treat breast cancer patients (Secretaría de Salud, 2011). Another fund, the Insurance for a New Generation, is also fully controlled by the CNPSS; it directly reimbursed in 2011 specialized providers for the treatment given to 33,688 children under five, for a total of US$ 8.4 million PPP (Secretaría de Salud, 2012). State health services limit their role in these two programs to referral of cases to providers previously certified by CNPSS.

Federal transfers to states attained the federation's policy aims of increasing net health expenditure for the non-insured, reducing the differences across states in their own levels of contributions, increasing per capita state contributions overall, and reducing the gap at the state level between the per capita expenditures of the insured and the non-insured. Total public health expenditure (federal plus state) on the non-insured went from 0.9 per cent of GDP in 2000 to 1.4 per cent in 2010. Federal health expenditure grew from 0.8 per cent of GDP in 2000 to 1.1 per cent in 2010, while state government contributions increased from 0.1 per cent of GDP to 0.3 per cent. Total health financing in terms of state GDP in 2000 ranged from 1.8 per cent in Querétaro to 5.0 per cent in Tabasco. States such as Estado de Mexico increased state expenditure by 105 per cent (at constant pesos), while others such as Campeche reduced spending by 70 per cent.

Total public health expenditures for health services to the non-insured showed an increase of 114 per cent (at constant pesos) between 2000 and 2010. Federal health contributions to state providers for the non-insured increased by 105 per cent in the period, while state contributions increased by 162 per cent.

Generally, financing was decentralized in relative terms insofar as the states had a greater increase, although it was not sufficient to significantly reduce their dependence on federal funding. The state with the smallest increase in total public health expenditure for the non-insured was Sonora, with 36 per cent, while the state with the greatest change was the Estado de Mexico, with 385 per cent. The state with the greatest federal funding increase (490 per cent) was Distrito Federal, while the state with the lowest federal increase was Baja California Sur (37 per cent), more than ten times the difference. Changes in state government contributions to health expenditure during the same period showed even greater variation, from a negative 68 per cent per person; this figure increased to 67 per cent in 2010. This change was brought about through more than doubling both the federal and the state budget for the non-insured, accounting for an increase from US$180 PPP in 2000 to US$385 PPP in 2010.

In the same period, the budget for social security institutions increased by 48 per cent. The closing of this gap was heterogeneous from the perspective of individual states: In the Estado de Mexico the gap was actually reversed: in 2010, for every dollar spent on an insured person, US$1.6 was spent on a non-insured person. In Aguascalientes, in contrast, the gap increased.

In general, closure of the gap between the insured and the non-insured gave ministers of health greater power to negotiate with social security institutions for the delivery of health care. Indeed, social security institutions often complained that privileges for their own beneficiaries were reduced, leading them to be more open to selling services to the wider population.

Governance

REPSS played an important role in transferring financial resources from the federal government to state providers. However, REPSS were constrained in their capacity to allocate resources with autonomy given their status as administrative organs of the state provider OPDs in most cases. In two exceptional states – Morelos and Baja California – REPSS were created as OPDs in themselves, although still reporting directly to the state ministries of health. Indeed, in these two cases the health provider OPDs are also independent from the state ministries of health. The capacity of REPSS to allocate funding to private providers or to fund public providers based on need and on performance were thus limited. Furthermore, REPSS receive their funding from the federal government with clear earmarks for line-item expenditures, further limiting their capacity to allocate resources. However, the experience of REPSS in states such as Hidalgo suggest they have a wider decision space. Indeed, in this state REPSS funds private providers using diverse contract types and a range of payment formulas such as capitation for primary care and case-based payment for hospital care. In this way, REPSS have introduced a modicum of competition with the intention of improving performance across the provider network, suggesting that leadership by state ministries of health is indeed a key factor to allow REPSS to exert their full potential.

Expenditures for non-personal health services were further earmarked by a program from 2009 through yearly Agreement for the Strengthening of Public Health Actions by the States (AFASPE). AFASPE transfers directly to the OPD or to the state treasury (depending on the origin of the funds with the AFASPE) the earmarked funding for public health for the whole state population, as well as the 20 per cent earmark for public health assigned by Seguro Popular to its affiliates.

The AFASPE agreement was designed to perform as a mechanism to coordinate diverse funding sources and to align them to specific preventive health care and health promotion programs at the state level, all according to explicit goals and timetables, accountability mechanisms, and process and impact indicators (Fundar, 2010). By joining the budgets for Seguro Popular affiliates and non-affiliates, AFASPE was meant to bridge diverse financial programs. While AFASPE aspires to be a performance-based funding mechanism, funding is set according to pre-established goals and not against attained targets. Furthermore, the Ministry of Health has not succeeded in transferring AFASPE funding in a timely manner nor in fully auditing expenditures. The Superior Federal Auditors – a congressional body – noted important unspent surpluses and expenditure delays amounting to 85 per cent of the total AFASPE for 2010 (Fundar, 2011). Another limitation of AFASPE is that Seguro Popular does not sign the agreements, and its funding commitment is thus in question.

In spite of the constitutional reform in the 1980s and the reform to the General Health Law in 2003, social security as represented by IMSS and ISSSTE remained fully segmented from the Ministry of Health as a federal provider as well as at the state level. The governance of social security in Mexico and of the almost half the population in the formal economic sector under its responsibility has been the exclusive prerogative of the federal government, with the exception of state and municipal bureaucrats who depend on state social security arrangements. This has led some policymakers to conceive of a dual system of social security for the formal sector and of social protection in health for the informal sector (Levy, 2008), while others would prefer to have social protection in health as an all-embracing state policy (Frenk & Gómez, 2009).

Access Rules

Seguro Popular is voluntary and at the individual level today. However, affiliation was originally at the household level, following the social security affiliation model. Individualization was introduced to stem the perverse incentive of state authorities to affiliate individuals within households as separate families and thus to increase their per-family contributions, a situation that threatened the capacity to attain universal coverage during the 2009 crisis. In a way, then, individualization reduced the states' decision space. Affiliation has no set periods as long as it occurs prior to the patients being discharged from hospitals if applications are made at the point of care. The federation constrains re-affiliation every three years. There are no pre-existing health conditions, although services are limited to the basic package of primary and hospital interventions and the high-specialty, catastrophic-cost interventions such as cancer care.

Hospitals and health centres have to be accredited by Seguro Popular before the REPSS are allowed to start affiliation of the population within their coverage area. REPSS were also given yearly affiliation quotas so the federation could gradually increase funding for the program. REPSS and OPDs were free to identify the priority population groups for affiliation and re-affiliation. States were also able to apply diverse criteria and technical resources for targeting population groups (Orozco et al., 2011). However, most states affiliated first the extreme poor, who were already covered by the cash-transfer program Prospera and for whom detailed lists of affiliates were at hand. This population was also mostly covered in twenty states through the IMSS Prospera program and its usually better-off health infrastructure. Access rules to Seguro Popular are therefore fairly decentralized, though constrained by broad federal rules.

Human Resources

Seguro Popular gave state health authorities an increased decision space given that they were allowed to hire personnel in direct relationship to patients in order to meet the increased demand from affiliates. The decision space for human resources hiring was moderate: contracting was specified as only for professional services without benefits, avoiding physicians finishing their studies and providing social service. Under this new scheme, hiring couldn't take place through permanent civil services payrolls, and new hires had to be in direct contact with patients, disallowing administrative, research, and planning hire. States had autonomy to hire for those services they considered most in demand. Today up to 70,000 employees – about 34 per cent – are directly managed by state ministries of health through this modality.

New hires have no social benefits and, until recently, accepted half the salary for equal work. To remedy this politically sensitive situation, the federal government first offered to integrate the entire workforce to federal posts. However, the economic crisis of 2009 pre-empted this, leading the Ministry of Health to order state governments to equalize salaries through the 40 per cent earmark of Seguro Popular funds. This led state ministries to curtail new hires and caused staffing crises, particularly in the newly built hospitals that were, in any case, not aligned to federal infrastructure policies.

Decisions by state administrators over federal civil service posts have been highly curtailed. OPDs have limited conflict-resolution capacities, as state authorities cannot change pay scale, responsibilities, or assignments, nor can they hire or fire workers, except those hired through Seguro Popular contracts. While OPD directors have been delegated the right of appointment to federally funded posts, strategic human resources decisions depend on the tacit or explicit consent of federal authorities and trade unions. Indeed, trade unions have the right to approve or refute all Ministry of Health human resources decisions (Merino, 2003; SSA & SNTSSA, 2011). The lack of differentiation between the OPD and the state ministry of health and the low level of decision space assigned to states by the federation and trade unions have restricted the state governments' capacity to exert a broad stewardship function over human resources and their influence on population health (Arredondo, 2003; Homedes & Ugalde, 2008; Orozco et al., 2011).

Organization Forms

Decentralization from the 1980s up until Seguro Popular was established did not alter in any meaningful way health services organization at the state level. Constraints in the ownership of infrastructure and especially in the hiring of human resources have stifled organizations within a traditional public sector and hospital-centred infrastructure. However, efforts have been made to improve the network of services at local levels through building small hospitals or health centres with greater capacity to address health needs, as well as through normative efforts to network the federal tertiary hospital infrastructure with the state secondary and primary care. Private providers are seldom used, as already stated, although private hospitals are now being contracted to tend to so-called catastrophic interventions.

Since the National Health Law gives responsibility for effective drug purchases, distribution, and dispensation to the state REPSS, state governments have had a wide degree of autonomy in this strategic area and have experimented with different approaches, including extending their public integrated systems, creating deconcentrated public agencies, and contracting out with private agencies. For contracting out, states have tried diverse formulas, going from a focus on purchase and distribution all the way to insourcing pharmacies within state hospitals or providing vouchers to purchase needed drugs in private pharmacies. A boom in private pharmacies selling generics and offering basic medical care today accounts for 16 per cent of total medical outpatient services in the country, putting pressure on public health authorities to reduce waiting times and to provide medications on demand.

Seguro Popular affiliation has now become the only mechanism envisioned to attain universal coverage for the non-insured. This has led states to affiliate all of the mostly indigenous, rural population already covered by the program IMSS-Oportunidades, despite the fact that this mostly poor population had free access to a wide package of health services. Affiliation of this population to Seguro Popular triggered financing by the CNPSS to state ministries of health through the established channels, opening to them the possibility of funding directly the IMSS-Oportunidades providers through contractual arrangements. Yet the new funding was not followed by a reduction in the transfers from the Ministry of Finance to IMSS-Oportunidades, nor in the funding that this program receives directly from the IMSS contributory fund. Indeed, elimination of the latter would imply a change to the IMSS law by Congress, something that has not been considered. Given the legal impasse and duplication of funding, state ministries of health have not yet established purchasing agreements with IMSS-Oportunidades and have limited their collaboration to traditional arrangements, aiming to delimit population coverage territories so as to ensure the efficient provision of services. Evidence from the state of Chiapas suggests that the affiliation of the IMSS-Oportunidades population to Seguro Popular and the strengthening of Ministry of Health infrastructure are in fact leading to a reduction in demand of IMSS-Oportunidades hospital services and an increase in those of the Ministry of Health.

Conclusions

Mexico remains a highly centralized country in spite of efforts from the early 1980s to devolve power to the states as a means of ensuring greater coordination of efforts towards development, poverty alleviation, and the effective operation of integrated disease control programs and primary health care. State ministries of health catering to the non-insured and to public health programs are highly centralized for both fiscal and human resources. Social security institutions are segmented, with various public agencies wielding central power over strategic decisions for the distribution of resources to cover specific social groups, while at the same time funding and providing their own services. This situation limits the role of state authorities to coordinate the health sector for equity, quality, and efficiency.

The health reform launched in the early twenty-first century with the introduction of the System of Social Protection in Health; its aim was to protect households without social security from catastrophic health expenditures and to bridge the gaps in health expenditure between the rich and poor Mexican states. New federal funding provided state health and REPSS authorities with greater capacity for deciding not only how and where to spend, but also which public or private providers to hire, inter alia, for the purchase and distribution of medicines (Orozco et al., 2011) and how many and what types of human resources to employ. Their control over local expenditures was curbed only by federal guidelines on budget cut-offs per object of expenditure (medicine, human resources, etc.). As a result, state ministries of health are now better able to manage a network of public providers to attain higher levels of efficiency and equity. State authorities, however, have little capacity to influence the direction of policy on the ground, given their still small proportion of state funding vis-à-vis federal contributions and the strict federal expenditure guidelines they are required to follow.

The federation, for its part, has strengthened financial transfer mechanisms to allocate resources in increased quantities and with improved efficiency with respect to national health priorities and targets. State development indicators have become more important to determine more equitable resource allocations. However, the federation has to give states greater flexibility to use their resources to contract providers who are better able to cater to the poor in rural areas and to poor sectors in urban areas. Such a greater degree of choice requires improved accountability mechanisms.

Seguro Popular can be characterized as a decentralizing policy: it attempts to strengthen a devolved state organization in its capacity to affiliate the poor and uninsured to a scheme providing access to a generous health care package. The conditioning of federal funding to the attainment of affiliation targets and state matched funding, as well as the establishment of specific state organs for affiliation and resource allocation, was certainly a step in the direction of decentralization. In practice, however, only federal funds are actually transferred to the state ministries of health or the OPDs on the basis of the population affiliated, with state contributions being mostly directed to investments in infrastructure, poor coordination with overall policy. Furthermore, federal resources are tightly controlled through line-item limitations that are not related to performance indicators, save for agreements that direct part of the earmarked expenditures to public health programs. While AFASPE attempts to coordinate diverse federal funding streams to respond to state needs, financing by state governments for public health programs is not required, promoted, or monitored. REPSS, for the most part, are dedicated to funding state health service providers given political pressures and a lack of capacity to contract private providers.

State health authorities have been given a much clearer role as executors of federal policy and have, to an extent, become more accountable. However, through earmarking resources, the federation places attention on process indicators and loses the capacity to benefit from the state authorities' position to identify and target local needs and to account for performance in attaining health objectives.

In spite of the intended strengthening of autonomy by state governments, their decision space was – by and large – decreased with Seguro Popular, precisely as a result of the administration of greater federal resources and the drive to affiliate the non-insured to attain universal health coverage – a federal policy. However, the actual decision space within states tends to vary, depending on the financial and human resource contributions by local governments and on the degree of innovation allowed by local politics. The contribution by state governments mostly through infrastructure investments places important demands on federal funding for human resources, supplies, and maintenance, thus implying a challenge to the federal decision space. With few additional federal resources now that universal coverage has been attained, state deficits may start to accumulate because the larger infrastructure will not be necessarily funded by the federation. This may increase pressure on state governments to fund current expenses, further increasing their decision space.

The new federal administration under President Enrique Peña Nieto has announced its intention to pursue universal health insurance, a policy that would imply greater coordination across federal social security agencies and with state ministries of health, as well as separation of financing and provision functions within all of them. Such a policy would require the development of the purchasing function – precisely the function that state REPSS were designed to perform. Universal health insurance may well imply greater power to state authorities for the coordination of Local Health Systems, as well as a greater role for national coordination and consensus mechanisms, such as that the National Health Council is now playing for the health sector.

REFERENCES

Arredondo, A. (2003). Federalismo y salud: Estudio de caso sobre el sistema mexicano de salud. In Foro de Federaciones, Instituto Nacional para el Federalismo, & Desarrollo Municipal (Eds.), *Federalismo y políticas de salud: Descentralización*

y relaciones intergubernamentales desde una perspectiva comparada (pp. 1–41).
Ottawa, ON: Forum of Federations. http://www.forumfed.org/libdocs
/Health01/120-HPFE110-mx-arredondo-s.pdf. Retrieved 11 September 2017.

Arredondo, A., & Orozco, E. (2006). Effects of health decentralization, financing and governance in Mexico. *Revista de Saúde Pública, 40*(1), 152–60.

Arredondo, A., Parada, I., Orozco, E., & García, E. (2004). Efectos de la descentralización en el financiamiento de la salud en México. *Revista de Saúde Pública, 38*(1), 121–9. https://doi.org/10.1590/S0034-89102004000100017

Arzoz, J., & Knaul, F.M. (2003). Inequidad en el gasto del gobierno en salud. In F.M. Knaul & G. Nigenda (Eds.), *Caleidoscopio de la salud: De la investigación a las políticas y de las políticas a la acción* (pp. 185–94). Mexico City, Mexico: Fundación Mexicana para la Salud.

Avila-Burgos, L., Cahuana-Hurtado, L., Montañez-Hernandez, J., Servan-Mori, E., Aracena-Genao, B., & del Río-Zolezzi, A. (2016). Financing maternal health and family planning: Are we on the right track? Evidence from the reproductive health subaccounts in Mexico, 2003–2012. *PLoS One, 11*(1), e0147923. https://doi.org/10.1371/journal.pone.0147923

Avila-Burgos, L., Cahuana-Hurtado, L., Pérez-Núñez, R., Aracena-Genao, B., & Hernández-Peña, P. (n.d.). El Sistema de Cuentas en Salud: Desarrollo, avances y retos – El caso mexicano. https://slidedoc.es/el-sistema-de-cuentas-en-salud-desarrollo-avances-y-retos-el-caso-mexicano. Retrieved 11 September 2017.

Brachet-Márquez, V. (2010). Seguridad social y desigualdad 1910–2010. In F. Cortés & O. de Oliveira (Eds.), *Los grandes problemas de México* (vol. 5): *Desigualdad Social* (pp. 181–210). Mexico City, Mexico: El Colegio de México.

Diario Oficial de la Federación. (1996, 25 September). Acuerdo nacional para la descentralización.

Frenk, J., & Gómez, O. (2009). La democratización de la salud en México. *Gaceta Médica de México 2001, 137*(3), 281–8.

Frenk, J., Lozano, R., & González Block, M.A. (1994). *Economía y salud, propuesta para el avance del sistema de salud en México, medición conjunta de días de vida sana perdidos por mortalidad prematura debida a enfermedad, accidentes o violencias y a tiempo de vida llevado con discapacidad o AVISA.* Mexico City, Mexico: Fundación Mexicana para la Salud.

Fundar. (2010). AFASPE: Presupuesto para programas de salud sexual y reproductiva. http://www.fundar.org.mx/mexico/pdf/SistemaProteccionSocialSalud.pdf. Retrieved 11 September 2017.

Fundar. (2011). Peo y contrape$o$ 2012. http://fundar.org.mx/peo-y-contrapeo -2012/. Retrieved 11 September 2017.

Gobierno de la República Mexicana. (1999). Quinto informe de gobierno. http://zedillo .presidencia.gob.mx/Informe1999/comuniesp.htm Retrieved 11 September 2017.

Gómez-Dantés, O., Sesma, S., Becerril, V.M., Knaul, F.M., Arreola, H., & Frenk, J. (2011). Sistema de salud de México. *Salud Pública de México, 53*(suppl 2), S220–S232.

González-Block, M.A. (1996). La descentralización de la Secretaría de Salud de México: El caso de los sistemas locales de salud 1989–1994. *Gaceta Medica de Mexico, 133*(3), 183–93.

González-Block, M.A., & Brown, A. (1997). Hacia la asignación equitativa de los recursos federales para la salud. In J. Frenk (Ed.), *El observatorio de la salud: Necesidades, servicios, políticas* (pp. 173–94). Mexico City, Mexico: Fundación Mexicana para la Salud.

González-Block, M.A., Leyva, R., Zapata, O., Loewe, R., & Alagón, J. (1989). Health services decentralization in Mexico: Formulation, implementation and results of policy. *Health Policy and Planning, 4*(4), 301–15. https://doi.org/10.1093/heapol/4.4.301

González-Block, M.A., Tapia-Conyer, R., & Olaiz, G. (1994). *Descentralización de los servicios de salud: El desafío de la diversidad.* Cuadernos de Salud 4: Organización y funcionamiento. Mexico City, Mexico: Secretaría de Salud.

Homedes, N., & Ugalde, A. (2008). 25 años de descentralización del sistema de salud Mexicano: Una experiencia para analizar. *Revista Gerencia y Políticas de Salud, 7*(15), 26–43.

Ibarra, I., Martínez, G., Aguilera, N., Orozco, E., Fajardo-Dolci, G.E., & González-Block, M.A. (2013). Capacidad del marco jurídico de las instituciones públicas de salud de México para apoyar la integración funcional. *Salud Pública de México, 55,* 310–17.

Levy, S. (2008). *Good intentions, bad outcomes: Social policy informality and economic growth in Mexico.* Washington, DC: Brookings Institution Press, University of Michigan.

López-Arellano, O., & Blanco Gil, J. (2008). Caminos divergentes para la protección social en salud en México. *Salud Colectiva, 4*(3), 319–33. https://doi.org/10.18294/sc.2008.348

Merino, G. (2003). Descentralización del sistema de salud en el contexto del federalismo. In F.M. Knaul & G. Nigenda (Eds.), *El caleidoscopio de la salud: De la investigación a las políticas y de las políticas a la acción* (pp. 195–207). Mexico City, Mexico: FUNSALUD.

Moreno, C. (2001). La descentralización del gasto en salud en México: Una revisión de sus criterios de asignación. Programa de Presupuesto y Gasto Público, CIDE y Fundación Ford. http://terceridad.net/PyPS/Por_temas/29_Gob_Fed/Decentr_GSM.pdf. Retrieved 11 September 2017.

Nigenda, G., González Robledo, L.M., Juárez, C., Sosa, S., Idrovo, A.J., Wirtz, V., . . . & Aguilar, E. (2010). *Evaluación de procesos administrativos del istema de protección social en salud 2009: Resumen ejecutivo*. Mexico City, Mexico: Instituto Nacional de Salud Pública.

Nigenda, G., & Ruiz, J.A. (1999). El caso de México. In Organización Panamericana de la Salud (Ed.), *Factores restrictivos para la descentralización en recursos humanos* (vol. 16) (pp. 151–79). Washington, DC: Programa de Desarrollo de Recursos Humanos.

Noriega, C., Huitrón, P., & Matamoros, M. (2006). Financiamiento al sistemas de salud en México. Working paper series: Innovaciones en el financiamiento de la Salud, No. 3 (52 pp.). Mexico City, Mexico: FUNSALUD-INSP. http://medicinaweb.cloudapp. net/observatorio/docs/rs/lg/Rs2006_Lg_noriega.pdf. Retrieved 12 September 2017.

Orozco, E., González-Block, M.A., Rouvier, M., Arredondo, A., & Bossert, T. (2011). *Evaluación, retos e innovaciones de la gestión de los regímenes estatales de protección social en salud para la cobertura universal*. Cuernavaca, Mexico: Instituto Nacional de Salud Pública.

Requejo, F. (2010). Federalism and democracy: The case of minority nations – a federalist deficit. In M. Burgess & A. Gagnon (Eds.), *Federal democracies* (pp. 275–98). London, UK: Routledge.

Romero-Martínez, M., Shamah-Levy, T., Franco-Núñez, A., Villalpando, S., Cuevas-Nasu, L., Gutiérrez, J.P., & Rivera-Dommarco, J.A. (2013). Encuesta nacional de salud y nutrición 2012: Diseño y cobertura. *Salud Pública de México, 55*(suppl 2), S332–S340. https://doi.org/10.21149/spm.v55s2.5132

Secretaría de Salud. (2011). *Boletín estadístico 2010: Número 30* (vol. 4). Mexico City, Mexico: Recursos Financieros.

Secretaría de Salud. (2012). Informe de resultados del SPSS 2011. Mexico City, Mexico.

SSA & SNTSSA. (2011). Condiciones generales de trabajo, 2011. https://es.scribd.com /doc/7625731/Condiciones-Generales-de-Trabajo. Retrieved 28 July 2012.

Soberón, G., Ruiz, C., Ferrando, G., Gomez, V., Laguna, J., Valadés, D., & Wit, G. (1983). *Hacia un Sistema Nacional de Salud*. Mexico City, Mexico: Universidad Nacional Autónoma de México.

World Bank. (2011). World development indicators database. http://siteresources. worldbank.org/DATASTATISTICS/Resources/GNIPC.pdf. Retrieved 12 September 2017.

Chapter Nine

Federalism and the Health System in Nigeria

OGOH ALUBO AND TEMITOPE AKINTUNDE

Structural Features of Nigeria

With a land area of almost 1 million square kilometers and a population of over 180 million, Nigeria is the largest and most populous country in sub-Saharan Africa. It is located in West Africa and comprises over 370 ethnic groups in thirty-six states and the Federal Capital Territory. It is also the eighth-largest oil producer and the fourth leading exporter of liquefied natural gas in the world. Nigeria's oil and natural gas resources are the mainstay of the country's economy, accounting for 96 per cent of total export revenue in 2012, according to International Monetary Fund (IMF) estimates.

Nigeria is a federation governed by the 1999 Constitution, which affirms that the country is one indivisible and indissoluble sovereign state (Federal Government of Nigeria, 1999), whose constituent units are bound together by a federal arrangement. It provides for a presidential system of government with three distinct, but complementary, branches: namely the executive, legislature, and judiciary, each acting as a check and balance on the powers of the other two. The Constitution further provides for the operation of three tiers of government, at the federal, state, and local levels.

The executive branch of government, at the federal level, consists of the president, vice president, and other members of the Federal Executive Council; at the state level, it is made up of the governor, deputy governor, and other members of the State Executive Council. There is also a legislature at the federal and state levels. The federal legislature, known as the National Assembly, is bicameral, comprising a 109-member Senate and a 360-member House of Representatives. At the state level, the legislature is known as the House of Assembly. The president, the governor, and their deputies, as well as members of the legislature at both federal and state levels, are elected for four-year terms; the tenure of the

Figure 9.1 Map of Nigeria showing the thirty-six states and the federal capital territory

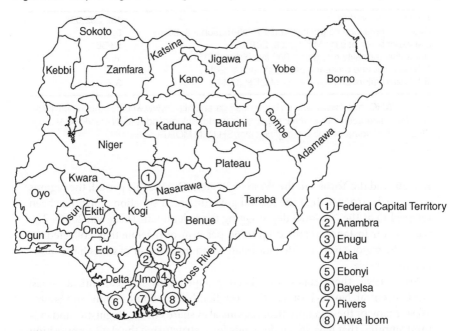

① Federal Capital Territory
② Anambra
③ Enugu
④ Abia
⑤ Ebonyi
⑥ Bayelsa
⑦ Rivers
⑧ Akwa Ibom

Source: Adapted from "Nigeria location map" by Uwe Dedering from Wikimedia Commons, licensed under CC-BY 3.0

executive officials is renewable only once. The tenure of members of the legislative arm may be renewed without limit. The local government legislative council is headed by the council chairman. Nigeria thus has a central government, thirty-six states (and the Federal Capital Territory), and 774 local government councils/areas whose operations are laid out in the Constitution. Some of its health characteristics are shown in Table 9.1.

Nigerian Federalism

Nature of Nigeria's Federalism

As a British colony, Nigeria was a unitary state until 1954, when it became a federation (Egwu, 2004; Elaigwu, 2005). At independence in 1960, Nigeria was a multi-ethnic state with separate regions dominated by three main ethnic groups: the Hausa-Fulani in the Northern Region, the Igbo in the Eastern

Table 9.1 Country indicators, Nigeria

Total population (2015)	182,202,000
Gross national income per capita (PPP international $, 2016)	5,740
Life expectancy at birth M/F (years, 2015)	53/56
Under-five mortality rate (per 1,000 live births, 2015)	109
Total expenditure on health per capita (intl $, 2014)	217
Total expenditure on health as % of GDP (2014)	3.7

Source: WHO, http://www.who.int/countries/nga/en/; http://www.who.int/pmnch/activities/ countries/nigeria/en/index1.html; https://data.worldbank.org/indicator/NY.GNP.PCAP. PP.CD; https://data.worldbank.org/indicator/SH.DYN.MORT

Region, and the Yoruba in the Western Region. During this period, the regions were much stronger than the federal government, a situation which has been referred to as the "regional dog wagging the federal tail" (Elaigwu, 2005). The regions, for instance, retained up to 60 per cent of revenue they collected. In 1967, the regions were divided into states, and the number of states has continued to increase.

Since 1996, these states have been grouped into six geopolitical zones: North-Central, North-East, North-West, South-East, South-South, and South-West. Many of these geopolitical regions also share ethnic, linguistic, and cultural affinities that have led to demands for restructuring the state composition of each zone, increasing the number of subnational units and responding to demands for self-determination of ethnic minorities (Elaigwu, 2005).

Nigeria has had long periods of military rule; the first coup in 1966 turned out to be the beginning of a series of coups, counter-coups, and coup attempts, and with these came rapid changes in leadership. When Nigeria celebrated its golden jubilee in 2010, a full twenty-nine of the fifty years of independence had been under military rule. The years of military rule experienced considerable centralization such that structures and institutions, which were hitherto controlled in the region or states, were brought under the control of the central government (Elaigwu, 2005; Nwolise, 2005).

The federal military government intervened often in the states, taking over schools, newspapers, and universities, and then moved responsibility for these activities to the federal legislative list. It also dissolved the regional police, creating a single Nigeria Police Force which remains (Alubo & Umar, 2011). By the return to democratic rule in 1999, the federation was more centralized than the more decentralized structures of the early postcolonial period. In effect, the states had been reduced to taking directives from the centre. These changes both in number of subnational units and in the relative centralization of authority at the federal level by the military governments have been described variously as "centralized federalism" (Elaigwu, 2005; Suberu, 2010) or as "a decentralized federal system with over-centralized concentration of power" (Okafor & Honey, 2004; Okojie, 2009).

Relationship between the Centre and Substate Structures

The relationship between the federal government and the states is guided by the Constitution. According to constitutional provisions, there are areas where the federal government has exclusive legislative authority, referred to as the "exclusive legislative list," and spheres where this jurisdiction is shared with the states, called the "concurrent legislative list." Most of the concurrent legislative list relates to infrastructure and social welfare such as housing, education, and health. The second schedule (part 1) of the 1999 Constitution (which was drawn up by the military) lists sixty-eight items on the federal exclusive legislative list. The concurrent legislative list defines the relationships between the "federation and the states," "among states and the federation," between "the states and the local government council," and "among the local government councils in the states" (Federal Government of Nigeria, 1999).

The separation of exclusive and concurrent lists enables the states to draw up their development plans and identify state priorities. Virtually all of the thirty-six states have development plans but also implement the agenda of the federal government. Periodically, the federal government draws up medium-term strategies such as the National Economic Empowerment and Development Strategy (NEEDS), which it mandates the states to implement as the State Economic Empowerment and Development Strategy (SEEDS) and lower down as the Local Government Economic Empowerment and Development Strategy (LEEDS) (National Planning Commission, 2004). All of these plans have health development content which the states are expected to implement.

One of the persistently problematic areas in the relationship between the federal government and the states is the control of resources and revenues. In the immediate postcolonial period, the formula was based on the concept of "derivation," in which more of the revenue was retained by the regions producing the resources, while factors such as population, land mass, and equality of states were also taken into account in the revenue-sharing formula (Dumoye, 2011). However, the formula was changed to "vertical allocation" by the military in 1967. Since then, income from all mineral resources such as oil is paid into a consolidated federal account and then disbursed to the states based on a formula that ensures that the federal government retains the lion's share of 48.5 per cent. The allocation formula is based on population and the amount of the state's contribution to the central purse through minerals and taxes. However, the central government keeps most of the revenues collected for its own uses. As a consequence, states and local governments constantly clamour for revenue sharing because they receive only 24 per cent and 20 per cent of federal revenue, respectively (Tyoden, 2001). These allocations from the centre are effectively the lifeline in most states because the funds account for between 46 per cent and 95 per cent of their annual budgets (Elaigwu, 2001).

Aside from the general complaint that the federal government has retained the largest share, there is also the sentiment that the majority ethnic groups that have historically dominated the federal government are shortchanging minority ethnic groups. There continue to be strident demands for fiscal federalism, which seeks to give states greater jurisdiction and control over resources located in such states.

While the current constitution provides for 13 per cent "derivation" for the states in the revenue sharing from the federation account, some are pressuring the federal government to increase that percentage. Using this principle, 13 per cent of oil revenues are earmarked and shared by the oil-producing states. State demands for a larger share of oil revenue have led to considerable conflict between the states of the oil-producing Niger Delta region and the federal government. This conflict has on many occasions taken international dimensions, with the emergence of ethnic militias engaged in pipeline vandalism and taking hostage foreign oil workers. More recently, Boko Haram, an Islamist movement in some states of the North-East zone which repudiates all forms of Western education and civilization, has engaged in armed struggle to overthrow the Nigerian state and pave way for a new one in accordance with its brand of Islam (Alubo & Umar, 2011).

The Health System

Nigeria operates a pluralistic health care delivery system with both formal and informal systems operating alongside each other. The private and public sectors and missionaries provide orthodox health care services in the country (Federal Ministry of Health, 2009). Although health is not in the concurrent list of the 1999 Constitution of the Federal Republic of Nigeria, in practice, all the tiers of government engage in different aspects of health care. Public health care provision in Nigeria is organized along the three tiers of government: the federal government provides tertiary care through the federal medical centres and teaching hospitals; the state governments provide secondary health care through the general hospitals; and the local government is largely responsible for primary health care provided through the primary health centres. The lack

Figure 9.2 Structure of the Nigerian health care system

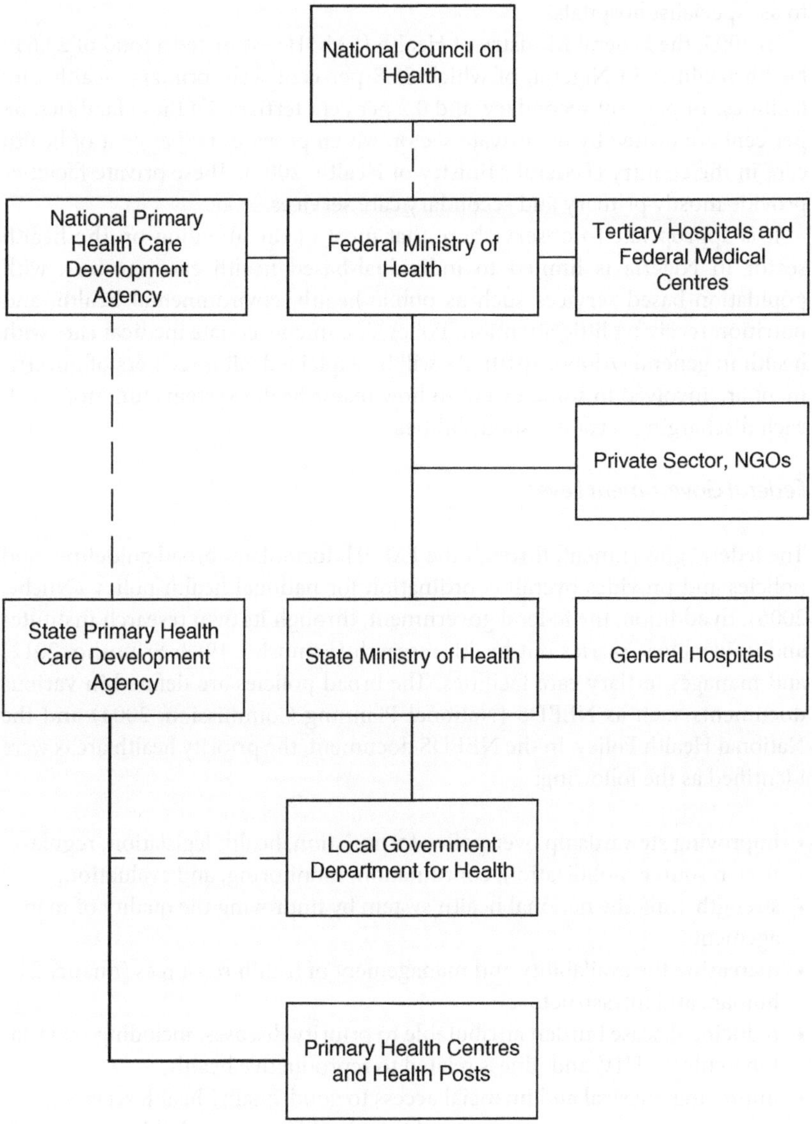

of clarity and specificity in the Constitution makes it possible for all tiers to engage in all three types of health care. Thus, many states which have universities run teaching hospitals; others also have tertiary facilities, mostly referred to as "specialist hospitals."

In 2005, the Federal Ministry of Health (FMOH) estimated a total of 23,640 health facilities in Nigeria, of which 85.8 per cent were primary health care facilities, 14 per cent secondary, and 0.2 per cent tertiary. Of these facilities, 38 per cent are owned by the private sector, which provides 60 per cent of health care in the country (Federal Ministry of Health, 2005). These private facilities provide mostly primary and secondary care services.

It is appropriate to observe here that most of the attention on the health sector in Nigeria is limited to individual-based health care services, with population-based services such as public health, environmental health, and nutrition receiving little attention. Policy documents equate medical care with health in general (Alubo, 2010). As will be explained, all three tiers of government are involved to some extent in how major health systems function, with each discharging certain responsibilities.

Federal Government Level

The federal government, through the FMOH, formulates broad guidelines and policies and provides overall coordination for national health policy (Nnebe, 2006). In addition, the federal government, through its own research institutes and universities, carries out health research (Erinosho, 1983; Erinosho, 2012) and manages tertiary care facilities. The broad policies are defined in various documents such as NEEDS (National Planning Commission, 2004) and the National Health Policy. In the NEEDS document, the priority health areas were identified as the following:

- improving stewardship over policy formulation, health legislation, regulation, resource mobilization, coordination, monitoring, and evaluation;
- strengthening the national health system by improving the quality of management;
- increasing the availability and management of health resources (financial, human, and infrastructure);
- reducing disease burden attributable to priority diseases, including malaria, tuberculosis, HIV, and illness related to reproductive health;
- improving physical and financial access to good-quality health services;
- increasing consumers' awareness of their health rights and obligations;
- fostering effective collaboration and partnership with all health actors.

These priorities of the federal government are also expected to be implemented by the states; in effect the former leads these initiatives while the latter models its efforts after the central government. The priorities identified in the National Health Policy are similar (Nnebe, 2006).

Coordination of national and state policy is the responsibility of the National Council on Health (NCH), an intergovernmental body chaired by the federal minister of health and made up of all state commissioners for health. This is made possible through the council of states structure, which exists for key ministries such as health and education. The NCH also has representatives from professional bodies, teaching hospitals, and the private sector. In this way, every tier of government as well as professional groups have the opportunity to debate and offer input into policy. In 2011, the NCH drew up a Strategic Health Plan for 2011–15 that was signed by the governors of all the thirty-six states (Federal Ministry of Health, 2010).

The federal government manages tertiary care hospitals such as university teaching hospitals and federal medical centres, which provide highly specialized services that for most Nigerians constitute the final stop in any episode of ill health. The teaching hospitals and federal medical centres also train various cadres of staff, including doctors and other health care workers.

The federal government coordinates a range of health targets such as maternal and infant mortality, immunization, and the drive towards the achievement of the health-related Sustainable Development Goals. It also runs special task forces in problem areas such as maternal mortality and immunization. In addition, the federal government runs drug control efforts through the National Agency for Food and Drugs Control (NAFDAC). NAFDAC is engaged in the uphill task of controlling the huge deluge of counterfeit drugs in the country (Alubo, 1993).

State Government Level

The State Ministries of Health (SMOH) are responsible for secondary hospitals and provide some regulation and technical support for primary health services within their jurisdiction. While they implement policies from the FMOH, each state may also formulate its policies to focus on local needs and priorities which may not be adequately reflected in the federal policy. In recent years, the federal policy of Primary Health Care Under One Roof has led states to establish State Primary Health Care Development Agencies or Boards. These agencies are responsible for the coordination and management of all primary health care (PHC) activities.

The public secondary health care facilities are run through the SMOH and its specific agency, the Health Services Management Board (HSMB). Each state

HSMB has a broad-based advisory committee comprising SMOH, HSMB, ministries for local government and education, non-governmental organizations, missionary facilities, and the private sector whose members are appointed by the state government (Nnebe, 2006). These facilities provide higher levels of care to patients and offer more specialized services in laboratory, diagnostic blood bank (for more complex investigation), rehabilitation, and physiotherapy (Nnebe, 2006). Many states also run tertiary facilities, the so-called state specialist hospitals.

Local Government Level

Primary health care is largely "the responsibility of the local governments with the support of the state ministries of health" (Nnebe, 2006, p. 232). PHC is promoted as the strategy for providing accessible health care services to the population and the fulcrum for health care development in the country. In accord with the concurrent legislative list, the states and local councils bear most of the responsibility of providing PHC. However, through the National Primary Health Care Development Agency (NPHCDA), a parastatal of the FMOH, the federal government still builds and runs PHC "model" centres in the local councils. Also, the State Primary Health Care Development Agencies work with the Local Government Areas (LGAs) to coordinate PHC services effectively.

As an entry point to the health care system, the PHC strategy was first attempted in the third national development plan period (1975–80) as the Basic Health Services Scheme but gained little actual implementation (Alubo, 1993). At its inception, the federal government led the way, with some international donor support, by building "model" PHC centres in some local councils. States were expected to learn from the models and replicate these in all local councils. In reality, however, the implementation "was haphazard and ineffective" and did not adequately cover the local councils (Achime, 1989; Kuti, 1988). PHC reform was re-launched by the federal government in 1986 and has since remained a cornerstone of Nigeria's health care system, albeit ineffectively implemented.

PHC services include routine consultations for common ailments, some laboratory investigations, and medications. PHC centres are run mostly by community health extension workers (CHEWs) and auxiliaries, rather than nurses and doctors.

Health matters at the local council level are coordinated by the LGA health committee chaired by the LGA chairman, while the medical officer of health or the PHC coordinator serves as the secretary of the committee. This committee is both an advisory and a coordinating body whose members are appointed by the state executive to represent broad interests, including local communities. The focus of PHC is largely dictated from the state through the SMOH and, increasingly in many states, the State Primary Health Care Development Agencies or Boards.

Health Care Budgeting and Financing

Like all other ministries, the budget for the Federal Ministry of Health follows several steps, beginning with proposals from the various units. Each federal hospital makes its own budget, submitted as part of parastatals of the FMOH. The various proposals are collated, discussed, debated, and passed on to the Budget Office. There are hearings at this level after which the budget is submitted to the presidency. All the submissions constitute the proposed budget for the federal government for the fiscal year. The annual budget for the federal government is then presented to the National Assembly. The budget goes through hearings in the National Assembly during which proposals may be modified. When all figures are agreed, the budget is passed into an appropriation bill for the fiscal year, which may sometimes extend to March of the following year instead of the normal January to December. The process usually involves lobbying, as figures could be retained, cut, or increased.

The appropriated sums are often higher than the amounts released. In the past decade, the difference, which is referred to as budget performance, hovers between 45 and 60 per cent of initial figures. This means that the medical care facilities are uncertain about how much money they would actually spend in any given year: budgets approved are rarely fully expended. Interaction in federal institutions and the state hospitals reveals that the situation is similar. In one of the federal facilities, capital projects which commenced in the 2009/10 fiscal year disappeared from the budget in 2010/11, leading to the stalling of the projects. This is a constant source of frustration as projects with a definite timeline linger after the due date.

In Nigeria, the major sources of health financing are through 1) the tax-based public sector that comprises local, state, and federal governments; 2) the private sector (including the not-for-profit sector), for which financing is done, directly or indirectly, through health insurance which employers purchase for their employees; 3) households, through out-of-pocket expenditures, including user fees paid in public facilities; 4) other insurance, social and community-based; and 5) external financing (through grants and loans) from donor organizations (Riman & Akpan, 2012).

Out-of-pocket expenditure is the major form of health financing, averaging 74 per cent of total health spending between 1998 and 2002, and represents a significant financial burden for households, preventing some from seeking care or resulting in financial catastrophe and impoverishment for those who do (Soyibo, 2009). There are no new figures of current health spending, but like most other aspects of consumption, it is likely to have increased.

Directly or indirectly, government budgets are financed mostly from oil royalty taxation supplemented by excise taxes, value added (sales) taxes, and sundry public fees. The Constitution mandates the federal government to keep a "federation account" for all revenues. Disbursements are made from this account to fund federal projects as well as fiscal transfers to the states.

State budgets are financed mostly through transfers from the federal government, commonly referred to as "statutory allocation from the federation account." Data on the percentage of state health care budgets which comes from federal transfers are not available. However, like the budget for other sectors, the estimates range from 70 to 80 per cent.

Funds to the local government councils come through the state government into the State Joint Local Government Account (Federal Government of Nigeria, 1999). This account is disbursed by the state governors to the councils, and often such disbursements may vary from actual transfers from the federal government to the local councils.

All three levels of care (primary, secondary, and tertiary) now charge fees for services and therefore have some internally generated revenue. These revenues, including drug revolving funds, in addition to statutory allocations, are used to support services.

According to a recent government document, between 2003 and 2005, total health expenditure (THE) increased by over 33 per cent. Within the same period, federal health expenditure rose threefold from N47.02 billion (US$293.8 million) in 2003 to N130.7 billion (US$816.9 million) and that of the states from N48 billion (US$300 million) to N78.8 billion (US$492.5 million) (Federal Ministry of Health, 2010). In spite of what these increases may suggest, the funding of health care has varied considerably and recently has declined significantly by comparative standards. Between 2003 and 2005, THE as a share of GDP declined from 12.25 per cent to 8.5 per cent (Federal Ministry of Health, 2010); and by 2010, THE had dropped to 5.1 per cent of GDP (World Bank, 2013), a much lower figure than the Abuja Declaration African leaders' consensus target of 15 per cent (World Health Organization, 2011).

Evolution of Health Sector Reforms

In recent years, as a consequence of the poor health system performance, the federal government has spearheaded a series of health sector reforms envisioned to drive improvements in service delivery and health outcomes. In 2003, the Health Sector Reform Program (HSRP), a document to cover 2003–7, was developed to kick-start this reform process. At the end of the period, it was noted that the HSRP was successful in helping the system to develop the required policy basis upon which a strategic agenda could be built.

The National Strategic Health Investment Plan (NSHIP) in 2007–8 succeeded the HSRP and was designed to articulate a strategic health development agenda geared towards achieving the Millennium Development Goals (MDGs), new international commitments for improved efficiency in health systems including the Paris Declarations, the International Health Partnerships, and the IHP+ Global Compact. The process for developing a National Strategic Health Investment Plan were initiated in 2007 and endorsed by the NCH in November of that year. However, considering the need to align the initiatives of the Federal Ministry of Health with other ongoing national development initiatives, the NSHIP was expanded and later developed into a National Strategic Health Development Plan (NSHDP).The NSHDP was designed to serve as the overarching reference document for actions in health by all stakeholders to ensure transparency and mutual accountability for results in the health sector (Federal Ministry of Health, 2009). Developed using a participatory bottom-up approach to ensure ownership by all the three tiers of government, it includes a framework to guide development of SHDPs at the different levels of government and a toolkit to ensure uniformity of federal, state, FCT, and LGA plans. The federal government, the thirty-six states, and the FCT each have an SHDP which seeks to address their respective priorities. In the end, the final NSHDP comprises the harmonized NSHDP and the individual federal, state, and LGA-level SHDPs and provides stakeholders with a global picture of the plan, its components, cost of implementation, and mechanisms for monitoring progress and ensuring successful implementation (Federal Ministry of Health, 2009). This framework has not guided health programming in the states and local councils as well as expected. For instance, de facto centralization in terms of the budget process and procurement of vaccines for immunization has continued in spite of supposed bottom-up orientation.

The National Health Act No. 8 of 2014

There have been concerted efforts to have a National Health Act to provide a framework for the regulation, development, and management of a national health system and to set standards for rendering health services in the federation. The National Health Bill, developed in 2000, eventually passed through several legislative delays and bottlenecks in 2012 and was signed into law in 2014.

The National Health Act was enacted to delineate and provide clarity to the roles and responsibilities of each tier of government, and to establish an organizational and management structure for the health system. It also is meant to strengthen PHC through improved provision for funding and management. For example, the act specifies that all Nigerians are entitled to a basic minimum package of health services (BMPHS). This package is a set of preventive, protective, promotive, curative, and rehabilitative health services or interventions, published from time to time by the minister of health after consultation with the National Council on Health.

To fund this BMPHS, the act establishes a Basic Health Care Provision Fund (BHCPF) to be financed from at least 1 per cent of the consolidated revenue fund of the federation, donor funds, and funds from other sources.

The act further specifies the disbursement distribution as follows: 1) 50 per cent of the fund shall be disbursed through the National Health Insurance Scheme (NHIS) and deployed towards the provision of the BMPHS in eligible primary or secondary health care facilities; 2) 45 per cent of the fund shall be disbursed through the NPHCDA and deployed to strengthening PHC services in eligible primary health care facilities (essential drugs, vaccines, and consumables; provision and maintenance of facilities; equipment and transport; development of human resources); and 3) 5 per cent of the fund shall be disbursed through a committee appointed by the National Council on Health and deployed towards emergency medical treatment (National Health Act No 8. 2014).

The act is yet to be implemented, as the Federal Ministry of Health is developing specific guidelines to govern the administration of the fund.

Decentralization and the Health System: Implications and Challenges

Despite (and often because of) the massive transformation and reorganizations in over fifty years of national independence, the Nigerian system of federalism is often denounced as a veritable source of, rather than a viable solution for, the country's multifaceted crises of poor governance, ethno-political conflict, and socio-economic underdevelopment (Suberu, 2010). One of the justifications for decentralization is that experience has shown that a highly centralized, top-down approach to service delivery is expensive, cumbersome, inflexible, and prone to abuse (Wunsch, 1999). In a country like Nigeria, where the majority of people live in rural areas and access care at primary health facilities closest to them, the argument becomes even stronger.

A distinct feature of the country's health care service and management is its decentralization at the three tiers and its attendant ambiguities (Ogunlela, 2011).

This decentralization policy that makes local governments run primary health care in Nigeria rests on the notion that services are most efficient when governance is close to the people (Abimbola, 2012). However, this has not been the Nigerian experience.

A strict interpretation of the Constitution of Nigeria with regard to the sharing of responsibilities between the three tiers of government implies that the state governments have the principal responsibility for basic services such as primary health and primary education, with the participation of LGAs in the execution of these responsibilities determined at the discretion of individual state governments (Gupta, Gauri, & Khemani, 2003). However, the constitutional existence of state-level discretion has contributed to disparities across local governments and states in the extent to which responsibility for primary health services is effectively decentralized. Moreover, the preponderance of primary health services and its adoption as the fulcrum for national health care delivery may explain the relative paucity of information on programs involving the secondary tier of care at the state level.

For example, the NSHDP affirms that to improve the health and well-being of Nigerians, the FMOH recognizes the need to scale up, strengthen the health systems including additional financing for health, and build and strengthen the primary health care system in line with the principles in the Ouagadougou and Abuja Declarations (World Health Organization, 2008). Furthermore, the NSHDP framework deals specifically with the organization of health services at the LGA level. Very little is written on state-level organization, yet states provide oversight functions for the activities of the LGAs which provide PHC, especially for rural dwellers.

The FMOH, however, strives to ensure state, as well as LGA, buy-in by making bottom-up participation an important component of its policy development and implementation processes. The development of the national strategic health plan, for instance, had representation from both states and LGAs in addition to other stakeholders. Also, the National Council on Health provides an avenue for state representation and input into policy decisions for health. Beyond this participatory approach, the states are mostly left to their own devices with the implicit understanding that health services in each state will be delivered within the overall policy context set by the FMOH. Furthermore, the flow of funds continues to be centralized, which in effect indicates that the bottom-up approach is yet to have much substance.

As an example of the latitude states have in terms of administration of health services, three states – Adamawa, Nasarawa, and Ondo – are currently piloting a novel results-based financing system for health service delivery in partnership with the World Bank. The states are making significant changes at the health centre level – introducing autonomy, enhancing management training, and offering financial incentives to centres that carry out pre-agreed services such as delivering babies safely and immunizing children, with due attention to quality. The objective is to reduce the obstacles commonly encountered at health centres, including low motivation among health workers, a lack of management, and frequent stock-outs of essential medicines and supplies (World Bank, 2012).

Some states have also created basket funds to finance priority health programs within their jurisdictions, while others have created State Primary Health Care Development Agencies to house all primary care delivery activities aimed at improving service delivery. The creation of SPHCDAs is a clear departure from the status quo ante where the LGAs run the PHCs with funding and supervisory support from the state.

Despite the challenges of the current system, opportunities for improvement exist, particularly with the National Health Act. Greater administrative and fiscal decentralization of services, many believe, will ensure that adequate health services are provided which meet the aspirations of the Nigerian people at all levels.

Decision Space Analysis

An overview of the current status of health services decentralization using the decision space analytic approach (Bossert, 1998) indicates that decision choices range from narrow to moderate and the degree of local input varies with the tier of government, as shown in Table 9.2. Perhaps because of the availability of more resources – human and financial – at the state level, more latitude is exercised here than at the LGA level.

Source of Financing and Resource Allocation

As indicated earlier, health expenditure and budgetary allocations at the state level depend on the own-source revenue capacity of each state. Typically, states and local governments receive financing from internally generated revenue and periodic allocations from the federation account. Sources of internally generated revenue, depending on the tier, include taxes, fines and fees, licenses, earnings and sales, rent received on government properties, interest repayment and dividend, and other miscellaneous revenue sources.

Transfers from the federal government are not earmarked. Each state and local government determines how they spend funds allocated to them. Based on revenue projections and sectoral priorities, each state draws up its budget and determines what percentage to allocate to different sectors, including health. Furthermore, they often provide budget and expenditure reports to the federal government.

Table 9.2 Summary of decision spaces in state and local governments in Nigeria's health system

Function	Indicator	Range of Choice		
		Narrow	Moderate	Wide
Financing				
Sources of revenue	Transfers from federal to state and to local councils		Fiscal transfers from the federal government account for a large proportion of revenue at state and local levels. But local own-source revenue varies considerably, so some states and local governments can decide to allocate more resources to health than other states and local governments.	
Allocation of expenditures	Proportion of funds earmarked by national authorities			Each tier determines to a reasonable extent the proportion of its revenue to allocate to health expenditures. There is no earmarking of funds transferred from the federal government except for specific programs.
Income from fees and contracts	Extent to which facilities can raise funds through user fees for services		Facilities can raise fees subject to approval of boards; approval is necessary before any expenditure from internally generated funds	
Fee schedule	Extent to which health facilities control fees charged and reviews		Proposed fees are presented to the boards for approval; same with reviews; expenses from all internally generated fees need board approval	

(Continued)

Table 9.2 Summary of decision spaces in state and local governments in Nigeria's health system (Continued)

Function	Indicator	Range of Choice		
		Narrow	Moderate	Wide
Service organization and delivery				
Hospital autonomy	Extent to which health facilities have control over services		Facilities may propose additions/revisions to services provided subject to approval by board or HSMB/SMOH	
Procurement	Extent to which state and local governments have control over procurement process and what is bought		All major procurements are as approved through local procurement process in federal hospitals and through SMOH/HSMB in state facilities	
Human resources				
Salaries	Differences in salary between facilities			Salaries for federal workers are determined by federal government salaries and wages commission, but states are not obliged to comply. States and LGAs set salaries for workers in their facilities through their respective service commissions. Federal salaries tend to be higher, leading to regular state workers' agitation for increases and/or strikes.

Contract employment	Extent of contract appointment for non-permanent staff	Conditions are as prescribed by federal government regulations, which states also implement
Civil service	Right of individual facilities to hire and fire	This is prescribed in the federal civil service regulations. Facilities seek approval from head of the service of the federation before employments can be made; disciplinary action can be taken locally but reported to board for ratification. In states, approval of the state civil service is required for employment; state hospitals can discipline.
Access rules		
Targeting	Defining priority populations	Access to health is guaranteed in the Constitution. States and LGAs, in a bid to improve access, can define and target specific population groups. Some states now provide free medical services to pregnant women, children under five years, and the elderly.

(Continued)

Table 9.2 Summary of decision spaces in state and local governments in Nigeria's health system (Continued)

Function	Indicator	Range of Choice		
		Narrow	Moderate	Wide
Governance rules				
State health care administration	Extent to which states are at liberty to set targets		States are obliged to implement federal targets but can set additional ones	
Local government	Nature of services and liberty to propose targets		Obliged to implement targets set at the state level but can notionally set own targets	
Hospital boards and health service management boards	Size and composition		Number and composition are determined by the federal ministry for federal facilities, and by state government for state facilities; same with HSMB	
Community participation	Number and composition of the community members and their roles		Number and who is involved are determined by the federal and state governments; roles are spelt out in federal and state regulations, but enforcement is weak so some local choice	

The federal government, therefore, does not have any significant influence on funds allocated to secondary and primary health care except those funded through special programs or agencies (World Health Organization, 2008). This scenario is also replicated downstream, with the state exercising little control over allocations by the local government. There is thus a high degree of autonomy in revenue allocation at both state and local government levels.

The size of statutory revenue allocation from the federation account, however, remains a major determinant of health care expenditure. It is expected that the measure of allocation received by state government from the federation account should also determine the amount of expenditure on health, with states that receive higher allocation from the federation account performing better (Riman & Akpan, 2012). In fact, there are significant variations in state revenues and health expenditure as a consequence of the vast majority of states depending heavily on revenue allocations from the federal government. In a World Bank study of decentralized delivery of primary health services in two states, it was observed that local governments in Kogi state are overwhelmingly dependent on statutory allocations from the federation account for their revenues and receive almost nothing from the state government. Revenue sources of local governments in Lagos are more diversified, with the bulk of their revenue coming from two sources, the federation account and the VAT (value added tax), but a significant amount is also internally generated from local tax bases. This is as one would expect given that Lagos state is the commercial nerve centre of Nigeria, while Kogi is a largely rural state (Gupta et al., 2003). The consequences for basic health service delivery between the two states are therefore clear – services in Kogi are more vulnerable to external shocks that affect oil prices and delays in release of allocation, which occasionally occurs. In recent times, there has been a steady move towards cost recovery, with the introduction of user fees at all tiers of government-owned hospitals. This has significant implications for access to service.

In conclusion, since the states and local governments depend largely on block grant intergovernmental transfers, but there is considerable variation of state or local contribution to health depending on own-source revenue, the decision space for financing ranges from narrow (with few local resources) to moderate (with significant local resources).

Governance

Institutional frameworks for health governance exist as guidelines prescribed at the national level to which states and LGAs must adhere. Secondary health facilities are managed by hospital management boards whose composition is stipulated in the National Health Policy. Specific appointments by the state governments are guided by these regulations.

State hospital management boards are responsible for the administration and management of the hospitals under their jurisdiction and ensure that the standard national guidelines for hospitals are implemented. Members include all health sector stakeholders (doctors, pharmacists, nurses, medical laboratory scientists, patients, etc.) and are appointed by the governor. The board is supervised by the state commissioner of health. As and when necessary, a state may, however, grant almost complete autonomy to individual hospitals and, in that case, the individual hospital boards, with wide representation, shall replace or complement the state organ (Federal Ministry of Health, 2004).

Similarly, governance of the PHCs involves structures such as ward and village health committees, whose members are drawn from the communities served by the health centres. These committees, whose membership is prescribed by national guidelines, play an important role in the coordination of planning, budgeting, provision, and monitoring of all primary health care services, though they are not always effective.

A major effort to introduce the concept of community co-management and co-financing of essential drugs as a strategy for improving maternal and child health through the improvement of quality of services in PHC facilities was found to be ineffective. An evaluation of the initiative in 2001 showed minimal evidence of community participation in drug management (National Primary Health Care Development Agency, 2001). Though designed to improve community participation, the national guidelines for setting up these committees are prescriptive, with definitions of the size, composition, and functions, which resulted in little or no efforts in the identification and strengthening of existing local social organizations, thereby causing a crisis of legitimacy (Federal Ministry of Health, 2009). The decision space will thus be considered moderate.

Access

As articulated in the National Health Policy, the objective is for all Nigerians, including those in remote areas, to have easy access to all levels of care. The thrust of the policy is the equitable distribution of health facilities to minimize risks, especially in underserved communities. Despite significant investments in health services, several barriers – geographical, physical, financial, and sociocultural – continue to limit access to health care. With 70 per cent of health expenditures still out of pocket, financial access to equitable health services remains a major challenge.

The reality of poor access is brought home by periodic health fairs organized by different groups including government agencies, at which services are provided "free" for a few days. These "fairs" are usually overcrowded – some indication that routine services are not easily accessible. This situation turns health care, which ought to be continuous, into a one-off encounter.

Free treatment (including food for hospitalized patients) was once provided in all facilities, federal and state, until the commencement of health reforms in the 1980s. Free treatment has given way to commercialization and cost recovery, all of them standard World Bank prescriptions (Turshen, 1999). These place some cost on services in the laboratory, as well as on drugs. This reform constitutes a huge burden, because in practice, service is denied those who cannot pay, and in case of hospitalization, deposits are required (Alubo, 2010). There are instances where patients who have recovered sufficiently to be discharged are held captive because of outstanding bills. Furthermore, service providers sometimes restrain themselves from requesting laboratory investigations that would normally be required. At the moment, the policy is implemented with little regard to ability to pay, particularly in the context of widespread poverty among the populace. To improve access, several state governments currently implement free health policies for priority demographic groups such as children, pregnant women, and the elderly.

The National Health Insurance Scheme, initiated in 2000, sought to reduce financial burden and improve access to health care. However, the scheme has concentrated on the formal sector of the economy, where employers pay premiums for their staff, and covers less than 2 million out of a population of 150 million (Federal Ministry of Health, 2010), almost all of whom are public-sector employees.

In addition to financial barriers, availability and distribution of functional health facilities and other health infrastructure continue to be variable across the country, with many public facilities being poorly equipped (Adeniyi, Ejembi, Igbineosun, & Mohammed, 2001). To address some of the infrastructure challenges, the federal government through the NPHCDA is involved in providing "model PHCs" at LGAs across the country. These model PHCs are well equipped and provide a minimum package of health benefits – the ward – which are a basic set of services to be provided by all PHCs. LGAs are also at liberty to implement infrastructural improvements, financial exemptions, and demand-generating activities which improve access to care within their jurisdictions. However, this is dependent on the leadership and level of political commitment available to follow through with these initiatives.

To improve access, state and federal subsidies help to minimize user fees through lower costs of drugs and overall policy of the Drug Revolving Fund

(DRF), which levies minimum drug costs to ensure restocking. In addition, childhood immunizations are fully subsidized by the federal government and free at public health facilities at all levels. Apart from immunization, states and LGAs exercise some level of discretion in defining and targeting specific population groups for increased access. Some states now provide free medical services to pregnant women, children under five years old, and the elderly. In terms of decision space analysis (Bossert, 1998), choices here are moderate since the LGAs generally follow the stipulated SMOH guidelines, which are tailored to reflect federal guidelines, as a baseline.

Human Resources Rules

There is currently a human resources for health (HRH) crisis in Nigeria, with widespread personnel shortages at all levels. Inadequate numbers of qualified health care providers, skewed distribution of available personnel in favour of urban areas, and migration (brain drain) to developed countries are some of the reasons for the current crisis. In recognition of the systemic deficiencies in the planning, management, and administration of available personnel, a National Human Resources for Health Policy (Federal Ministry of Health, 2006) and its corresponding Strategic Plan for 2008 to 2012 (Federal Ministry of Health, 2008) were developed. Interventions contained therein guide investments and decision-making in the planning, management, and development of HRH at the federal, state, LGA, and institutional levels.

The National Health Act, it is hoped, will address issues of human resources management within the national health system in order to ensure adequate human resources planning, development, and management structures at national, state, and local government levels, as well as availability of adequate resources for the education and training of health care personnel. The act empowers the minister of health in concurrence with the NCH to, among other things, develop guidelines that will enable the state ministries and local governments to implement programs for the appropriate distribution and training of health care providers and health workers, as well as to prescribe strategies for effective recruitment and retention of health workers within the national system.

Currently, salaries and emoluments for health care workers are determined at each tier of government by the responsible agency or commission. At the federal level, salaries are set by the Federal Salaries and Wages Commission, thus ensuring uniformity among employees of tertiary facilities. A similar structure governs salaries as well as recruitment at both state and local government levels, with each tier exercising its autonomous powers to hire, fire, and determine wages for its employees. However, all federal health facilities must obtain permission from the centre before any recruitment. These powers are exercised by the management boards, not the individual facilities. However, experience shows that there are agitations by health workers – and other workers – at state and local council levels for the same salary levels as the federal governments. These agitations have led to several strikes as state governments indicate lack of capacity to meet federal salary levels.

Since the purchasing power of the tiers is largely determined by their revenue capacity, the federal government typically pays higher salaries than the state and local governments. This has invariably contributed to the imbalance in the distribution of human resources for health. Primary health care facilities, particularly in rural areas, have worse manpower shortages: only 12 per cent of practicing doctors work in both public and private PHC facilities (Federal Ministry of Health, 2006). This operational framework can be construed as broad decision space for human resource management at both state and LGA levels.

Service Organization and Delivery

The decision space is largely narrow in terms of service delivery and organization from the facility perspective. Although individual hospitals are not autonomous, changes can be made to services provided with the approval of the management board. These changes, however, cannot be so radically different as to neglect provision of basic health services and priority programs defined in the national guidelines. Facilities have narrow decision space generally, as their activities are under the supervision of the HSMBs or the LGA authority. As such, service changes such as user fees are subject to the approval of the governing boards or authorities. The result is that states and LGAs (through their respective boards) exercise some degree of autonomy over service delivery decisions at individual facilities and thus decision space at these levels will be considered moderate.

Secondary facilities have some limited autonomy in purchasing drugs and minor equipment through the Drug Revolving Fund, which itself is a program of health sector reform. DRF is a scheme ensuring that proceeds from the sale of drugs to patients are placed in a special fund to enable restocking. Through the DRF scheme, each facility can routinely replenish drugs to ensure constant availability. Other drugs, as well as major equipment, are obtained through the procurement system of the HSMB. Capital projects (mostly construction and major renovations) are, however, carried out by the SMOH, mostly through tendering for contracts. Purchases by the HSMB as well as the SMOH are guided by the Public Procurement Act.

Conclusion

Although Nigeria has entrenched decentralization in its Constitution, the country's experience suggests that both state and local governments have failed to deliver public services, including health, in accordance with this principle (Okojie, 2009). As indicated in this chapter, constraints on effective fiscal and administrative decentralization are varied. There is general over-concentration of political and financial power as well as human resources at the federal level to the detriment of state and local governments. There are no clear guidelines on the interface between central line ministries and local governments. Thus, there remains a fundamental mismatch between account-ability and responsibility structures (Stokes-Prindle et al., 2012). Furthermore, decentralization has been used by ruling parties at the federal and state levels to renew or consolidate their power and influence governments at the local level. At the moment there is enormous centralization of the central govern-ment in relation to the states; the same is replicated between the states and local governments.

It is uncertain whether the current clamour for "true federalism," resource control, and secessionist campaigns by movements such as Boko Haram and Indigenous People of Biafra would lead to more overall decentralization. Fur-thermore, in March 2014, the federal government held a national conference of 492 persons representing various interests to debate a wide range of issues, including the nature of federalism. It is anticipated that these efforts would pave the way for greater and more effective fiscal and administrative decentraliza-tion, which could trickle down to the health system.

The National Health Act will result in restructuring of the administration and financing of the health system, albeit with less decentralization, particu-larly at the LGA level, than currently exists. However, it is hoped that the act, when implemented, will deliver on its intent of providing a more robust frame-work for improved delivery of health services in Nigeria.

REFERENCES

Abimbola, S. (2012). How to improve the quality of primary health care in Nigeria. Retrieved from http://blogs.bmj.com/bmj/2012/06/22/seye-abimbola-how-to-improve-the-quality-of-primary-health-care-in-nigeria/

Achime, N. (1989). Health sector in a developing country. *An Analysis of Primary Health Care in Nigeria Scandinavian Journal of Development Alternatives*, 8(4), 159–84.

Adeniyi, J.D., Ejembi, C.L., Igbineosun, P., & Mohammed, D. (2001). *The status of primary health care in Nigeria: Report of a needs assessment survey*. Abuja, Nigeria: National Primary Health Care Development Agency.

Alubo, O. (2010). In sickness and in health: Issues in the sociology of health in Nigeria. University of Jos Inaugural Lecture Series No. 41.

Alubo, O., & Umar, M. (2011). Nigeria and the challenges of national integration. In M. Maduagwu & A. Akpuru-Aja (Eds.), *Nigeria's 50 years of nation-building: Stock-taking and looking ahead* (pp. 107–30). Kuru, Nigeria: National Institute.

Alubo, S. (1993). Implementing health for all in Nigeria: Problems and constraints. In P. Conrad & E. Gallagher (Eds.), *Health and health care in developing countries* (pp. 228–45). Philadelphia, PA: Temple University.

Bossert, T. (1998). Analyzing the decentralization of health systems in developing countries: Decision space, innovation and performance. *Social Science & Medicine, 47*(10), 1513–27. https://doi.org/10.1016/S0277-9536(98)00234-2

Dumoye, A. (2011). Nigeria's constitutional development in perspective. In M. Maduagu & A. Akpuru-Aja (Eds.), *Nigeria's 50 years of nation-building: Stock-taking and looking ahead* (pp. 43–66). Kuru, Nigeria: National Institute.

Egwu, S. (2004). Beyond "native" and "settler" identities: Globalization and the challenges of multicultural citizenship in Nigeria. In J. Moru (Ed.), *Another Nigeria is possible*. Abuja, Nigeria: Nigeria Social Forum.

Elaigwu, I. (2001). Military rule and federalism in Nigeria. In I. Elaigwu & R. Akindele (Eds.), *Foundations of Nigerian federalism* (pp. 166–93). Jos, Nigeria: IGSR.

Elaigwu, I. (2005). *Nigeria yesterday and today for tomorrow*. Jos, Nigeria: Aha Publishing House.

Erinosho, O. (1983). Health planning in Nigeria. *Nigerian Journal of Sociology and Anthropology, 8*, 34–49.

Erinosho, O. (2012). Some thoughts on accountability in, and responsibility for health in Nigeria. *Quarterly Newsletter of the Health Reform Foundation of Nigeria, 1*(1), 1–5.

Federal Government of Nigeria. (1999). *Constitution of the Federal Republic of Nigeria*. Lagos, Nigeria: Government Printer.

Federal Ministry of Health. (2004). Revised national. *Health Policy (Amsterdam)*.

Federal Ministry of Health. (2005). Inventory of health facilities in Nigeria.

Federal Ministry of Health. (2006). National Human Resources for Health Policy.

Federal Ministry of Health. (2008). National Human Resources for Health Strategic Plan 2008–2012.

Federal Ministry of Health. (2009). National Strategic Health Development Plan framework (2009–2015).

Federal Ministry of Health. (2010). National Strategic Health Development Plan 2010–2015.

Gupta, M., Gauri, V., & Khemani, S. (2003). Decentralized delivery of primary health services in Nigeria: Survey evidence from the states of Lagos and Kogi. Development Research Group, World Bank Africa Region Human Development Working Paper Series.

Kuti, O. (1988). Speech at the opening of national conference on the problems of rural dwellers at National Institute of Policy and Strategic Studies. Kuru, Nigeria.

National Planning Commission. (2004). *National Economic Empowerment and Development Strategy*. Abuja, Nigeria: National Planning Commission.

National Primary Health Care Development Agency. (2001). Evaluation of the Bamako Initiative.

Nnebe, H. (2006). *National Health Policy P219-274: Policies of the Federal Republic of Nigeria 1999-2007*. Kaduna, Nigeria: Joyce Graphics.

Nwolise, O. (2005). How the military ruined Nigeria's federalism. In E. Onwudiwe & R. Suberu (Eds.), *Nigerian federalism in crisis: Critical perspectives and political options* (pp. 114-26). Ibadan, Nigeria: Programme on Ethnic and Federal Studies.

Ogunlela, Y. (2011). An appraisal of Nigeria's health sector and its healthcare delivery system. *Journal of Food, Agriculture and Environment, 9*(3&4), 81-4.

Okafor, S., & Honey, R. (2004). Oil and territorial decentralization in Nigeria. *African Geographical Review, 23*(1), 5-22. https://doi.org/10.1080/19376812.2004.9756176

Okojie C. (2009). Decentralization and public service delivery. International Food Policy Research Institute. Nigeria Strategy Support Program (NSSP) Background Paper No. NSSP 004.

Riman, H., & Akpan, E. (2012). Healthcare financing and health outcomes in Nigeria: A state level study using multivariate analysis. *International Journal of Humanities and Social Science, 2*(15), 296-309.

Soyibo, A. (2009). *National health accounts (NHA) of Nigeria*. Abuja, Nigeria: Federal Ministry of Health.

Stokes-Prindle, C., Wonodi, C., Aina, M., Oni, G., Olukowi, T., Pate, M.,, ..., & Levine, O. (2012). *Landscape assessment of routine immunization in Nigeria: Identifying barriers and prioritizing interventions*. Baltimore, MD: International Vaccine Access Center.

Suberu, R. (2010). The Nigerian federal system: Performance, problems and prospects. *Journal of Contemporary African Studies, 28*(4), 459-77. https://doi.org/10.1080/025 89001.2010.512741

Turshen, M. (1999). *Privatizing health services in Africa*. New Brunswick, NJ: Rutgers University Press.

Tyoden, S. (2001). The minorities factor in Nigerian federalism. In I. Elaigwu & R. Akindele (Eds.), *Foundations of Nigerian federalism* (pp. 246-65). Jos, Nigeria: IGSR.

World Bank. (2012). Three Nigerian states inject new life into healthcare for mothers and children. http://web.worldbank.org/WBSITE/EXTERNAL/COUNTRIES/AFRI

CAEXT/0,,contentMDK:23169752~menuPK:2246551~pagePK:2865106~piPK:2865
128~theSitePK:258644,00.html. Retrieved 29 August 2017.

World Bank. (2013). Health expenditure, total (% of GDP). https://data.worldbank.org
/indicator/SH.XPD.TOTL.ZS. Retrieved 29 July 2013.

World Health Organization. (2008). Ouagadougou Declaration on Primary Health
Care and Health Systems in Africa: Achieving better health for Africa in the
new millennium. http://ahm.afro.who.int/issue12/pdf/AHM12Pages10to21.pdf.
Retrieved 8 September 2017.

World Health Organization. (2011). The Abuja Declaration – ten years on. http://www
.who.int/healthsystems/publications/Abuja10.pdf. Retrieved 29 July 2013.

Wunsch, J. (1999). Institutional analysis and decentralization: Developing an analytical
framework for effective Third World administrative reform. In M.D. McGinns (Ed.),
Polycentric governance and development (pp. 243–68). Ann Arbor, MI: University of
Michigan Press.

Chapter Ten

Conclusion: An Overview of Eight Federal Country Case Studies of Health System Decentralization

THOMAS J. BOSSERT AND GREGORY P. MARCHILDON

Introduction

This collection of eight important cases of federalism and the health sector in different countries gives us a significant range of experiences in federalism and health system decentralization. As noted in other recent comparative studies, the cases presented here show that far from being simple categories, federalism and decentralization are complex and varied administrative and political structures, with considerable variation within the categories (see also Costa-Font & Greer, 2013; Fierlbeck & Palley, 2015). However, there is an important connection in that, relative to unitary states, the formal separation of powers stipulated in at least some federal constitutions can bestow on subnational jurisdictions greater authority over, and responsibility for, the public funding, regulation, and management of the health sector. At a minimum, the intergovernmental institutions and processes more generally associated with federations than with unitary states highly influence the institutions and instruments used by subnational governments in the health sector.

Federalism and Constitutional Assignment of Roles and Responsibilities

Federalism is a constitutionally determined administrative and political structure (Marchildon, 2009). The constitutions in this set of cases have defined the role in the health sector of the central (often called the federal or national) government and those of the subnational governments in a wide variety of ways. Constitutions in some countries (South Africa, Brazil, Mexico) define specific roles for each level and in others (Pakistan, Nigeria, Germany, Switzerland, South Africa) grant authority and responsibility to several levels in "concurrent lists" of functions that are either shared or parallel in implementation. In some cases (Switzerland, Germany, South Africa, Nigeria), the authors have often had to give significant background about the general federal structure before discussing the specific application to health, while others (Pakistan) have constitutional items or amendments focused directly on health sector issues.

The bulk of the constitutional decentralization in some countries (Canada, Mexico, Switzerland) assigns responsibilities to the state, province, or canton levels; in others specific responsibilities are also assigned to the next levels down, usually municipalities, districts, or counties (Switzerland, Brazil, South Africa, Nigeria). In these cases there is a competitive tension among the subfederal levels, with some countries (such as South Africa and Mexico) having strong provincial or state authorities which limit the lower levels to very narrow decision space. Brazil is an exception which by constitution assigns the major responsibility for health to the municipalities and sees the state and federal levels in a supporting role. However, in practice the Unified System restricts the decision-making power of Brazilian municipalities.

It is also important to examine the effects of federalism when it grants more decentralization to the first subnational or regional level of governance (e.g., provinces or states) than to more local levels (e.g., districts or municipalities) of governance. For instance, in Pakistan, the constitutional amendment granting significant devolution to the provinces has resulted in a recentralizing of authority from the districts to the provinces. Although not covered in this volume, India offers an example of how a constitutional amendment has encouraged states to decentralize to substate levels (block, village) even while allowing each state to determine the degree, the process, and the timing of this decentralization.

Some constitutions have required forms of citizen participation in addition to the state, provincial, or local governments. Brazil's constitution requires civil society health councils with more than advisory power at all three constitutional levels of government.

The "right to health" in both Mexican and Brazilian constitutions acts as a vehicle for federal involvement – some would say interference – in subnational states and municipalities. Similarly, the federal spending power and standards of coverage for medically necessary services in the Canada Health Act function as a constitutional means of limiting provincial decision space. Although in Switzerland the constitution explicitly makes health an individual responsibility, since it contains a constitutional commitment to equity and it requires both central and cantonal governments to ensure that individuals have economic protection against illness and old age, it offers some ground for central responsibility. In Germany, the constitutional commitment to "uniform living conditions" may function in a similar way by establishing uniform rights across the different states. In South Africa, the constitution allows the federal level to intervene in provincial and municipal health governance if the provinces are not achieving national policy norms, if another province is endangered, or for national security issues.

There do not seem to be clear differences in the way decentralization in health is structured based on whether a country's governments are organized in a presidential system (Brazil, Mexico, Nigeria), a parliamentary system (Germany, Canada, Pakistan), or a mix of these two main systems (Switzerland, South Africa).

What does seem common in federal systems is the importance of coordinating mechanisms among non-federal governmental health ministers. These mechanisms include the Mexican Board of Health (which convenes the state health ministers quarterly), the Brazilian Tripart Intergovernmental Commission (CIT), the Swiss Conference of the Cantonal Ministers of Public Health (CCMPH), the Nigerian National Council on Health, and the Conference of Federal/Provincial/Territorial Ministers of Health in Canada. These are usually advisory bodies that provide a forum for interaction and sharing information. In most cases, these are not bodies that can make binding decisions; however, the Swiss CCMPH is able to sign binding "treaties" with the Confederation. Switzerland also has created "horizontal" regional mechanisms of coordination combining several cantons, each of which has its own administrative structure and financing.

There is an unusual situation in Germany where some functions are held at the national legislative level but the state governments, collectively, have a veto over changes in legislation in one house of the legislature – the Bundesrat. Depending on the political party that dominates the Bundesrat, this can prevent the federal executive from achieving its health policy reforms.

It is also important to consider the historical evolution of federalism – as an extreme case, in Germany the states were independent before the federal government was created and, indeed, the creation of the welfare state and social insurance was part of a long historical process of strengthening the central government. Other nations were formed as federal states at the end of colonial periods that established the nation-state (Mexico, India, Pakistan, Nigeria) or in a more gradual evolution to self-government (Canada). Switzerland and South Africa may be something in between, with fierce cantonal and linguistic identities in Switzerland and the apartheid fragmentation of townships in South Africa. Nigeria's federalism is also based on the recognition of the geographic domination of distinct ethnic groups.

Political Economy and Capacities

Recent studies in political economy and comparative policy analysis suggest that the characteristics and effectiveness of different approaches to federalism and decentralization may be influenced by the political economy and especially how it shapes the system capacities (Tuohy, 2009). The cases reviewed here span a wide range of different political economy characteristics, from low-middle-income Pakistan and Nigeria, to high-middle-income Brazil, Mexico, and South Africa, to high-income Canada, Germany, and Switzerland. The role of market economy versus more state intervention may also influence the character of decentralization. Political economy approaches also include varieties of political systems even within countries over time: authoritarian military regimes in Nigeria and Pakistan; relatively authoritarian democratic systems such as Mexico under the PRI; varieties of parliamentarian systems in Canada, Germany, India, and Pakistan; and presidential regimes in South Africa, Switzerland, and Nigeria (Immergut, 1990). Recent literature on the role of corporatism as a governance structure may also influence federalist and decentralized systems (Acemoglu & Robinson, 2012).

With the small number of cases and this variety of political economy characteristics, it is not possible to draw definitive conclusions about the influence of these broad characteristics on the types of federalism and decentralization, nor on the possible influence they might have on health system outcomes.

However, we do find some characteristics of what we will call "capacities" at least potentially influenced by having differing levels of economic resources, different roles of the private sector, and different governing structures. The capacities required by subnational governments to carry out their responsibilities seem to depend on the income level in the country and on differences between regional and local governments. In particular, the capacity to take on greater decision space at state or provincial levels is not an issue in high-income countries such as Canada, Germany, and Switzerland. However, lack of capacity appears to be a major issue in lower-income nations, and lower administrative levels (municipal or district) seem to have more concerns about their respective capacities to assume more decision space. In South Africa, for example, the provinces clearly have greater capacities than do the districts to manage their health systems and have had more experience doing so. There is also a significant variation across South African provinces in terms of both administrative capacities and the relative level of corruption. A similar condition was found in Nigeria, where lack of local own-source revenues in many local governments significantly limited their capacity to implement health activities.

In some middle- and low-income countries, the capacities of the national ministries of health and other health agencies such as the social insurance agencies are also limited. In South Africa and Nigeria, the technical and managerial capacities at the national level are insufficient for managing a decentralized system. Fragmentation of health funding and provision, as illustrated by Mexico, can act as a further constraint in terms of subnational capacities.

In some countries (Mexico and Brazil), non-federal governments had to demonstrate capacities in order to gain additional decision space. In the first process of decentralization under the de la Madrid government in Mexico, only twelve states qualified in terms of technical staff and administrative capacity.

Corporatism

Corporatism in Mexico and in Germany, and to a lesser extent in Canada, is also an additional structure that may play an important role in decentralization. In Germany the meso-level semi-autonomous corporatist "peak" organizations, made up of the sickness funds and the providers, are delegated the responsibility to reach agreements on payments and coverage issues, in some ways replacing the role of the governmental line organizations at the state and local levels. In Mexico the corporatist structures of the dominant political party (the PRI) for decades structured the centralized health system. As democratization processes eroded the support for the PRI, openings for a more decentralized federation have encouraged greater decision space at the state level. In Canada the role of the provincial medical associations that negotiates with the provincial governments is a modified form of corporatism.

Fragmentation of Health System Actors

The fragmented financing institutions in some countries seem to have the effect of reducing some aspects of decentralization. For instance, in Mexico the large social insurance parallel system of IMSS is a major funder and provider of health services and is highly centralized. Another set of parallel structures in Mexico is the OPD (Decentralized Public Organizations), which manage federal block grants to the states, bypassing their state treasuries. Similarly the alternative funding sources for social health insurance schemes in Germany and Switzerland also fragment the control that is assigned to subnational governments. So while these subnational units have increasing formal control over the public tax-financed system, some of that control is eroded by these parallel structures.

Processes of Change in Federal Structures

It has long been recognized in some of the literature on federalism in the United States that the degree of local control follows a sequence of ebb and flow between the centre and the subnational units (Nathan, 1993). Perhaps the best case in this study is that of Mexico, which decentralized to some states in the 1980s, recentralized in the late 1980to the 1990s, and decentralized again in recent years. In Canada the experiments with regional authorities in different provinces also resulted in an ebb and flow of assigned responsibilities. The overall trend in Canada was an initial attempt at centralization at the federal level, followed by a long process of strengthening the provincial authority.

An example of another process of decentralization is the use of decentralization by democratic governments that follow centralizing military dictatorships. In Nigeria and Pakistan, the drive for increased decentralization was seen as an antidote to the military government and a part of the democratization process. Although not cases in this volume, the Philippines and Indonesia also experienced this pattern.

Introduction of Competition and Market Effects

States can create greater decentralization by replacing government programs and regulation with market-based mechanisms and private-sector actors. Indeed, governments have used privatization as a conscious strategy to achieve a greater level of health system decentralization (Atun, 2007). However, in the case studies presented in this volume, it was more common for governments to introduce reforms that mimic market effects rather than engage in outright privatization. Nevertheless, the Canadian, Brazilian, and Swiss systems have significant private-sector providers within public or social insurance financing systems.

The introduction of financing reforms in which money follows the patient rather than providing historically based budgets to facilities has had an important effect of reducing the control of both federal and non-federal levels. This is particularly true in systems where the patient can choose the location of services (as in Switzerland, where a patient can choose services in other cantons than his or her residence) or the type of service (private rather than public). South Africa, for example, is considering the creation of an insurance agency which will purchase services from both public and private facilities directly (without provincial or district involvement) and may pay according to the choice of patients.

Social Health Insurance

One of the most important institutional differences among countries is whether the state funds and provides health services directly or whether the state acts principally as a regulator of health insurance. The choice of these two policy instruments is determined by the political and social history of the country, as illustrated by the evolution of social health insurance (SHI) from its Bismarckian origins in the late nineteenth century (Saltman & Dubois, 2004).

While often not a constitutionally assigned role (except in Switzerland, which assigns the role exclusively to the federal government), the role SHI institutions play is another complicating factor in assessing the decision space of both the federal and non-federal governments. Although tax revenue either from the federal treasury (as in Germany) or from the enforced cantonal subsidy in Switzerland is part of the SHI funding, the major source of funding comes from non-governmental SHI funds, which in general reduces central government control. Mexico has a combination of funding sources including earmarked major tax transfers and a separate autonomous social insurance agency. This issue is likely to become more important as SHI countries attempt to implement a policy of universal insurance coverage for all of the population, as promoted by the World Health Organization.

This issue is becoming more important as both South Africa and Mexico are discussing the introduction of National Health Insurance (NHI) in a way that introduces a major split between those holding the funds as a separate payer and the decentralized governments as organizers of providers. In addition, Nigeria has just started a social insurance program mainly for public-sector formal employees which may be expanded to a larger portion of the population.

Decentralization: Decision Space Framework

As noted in the introduction, the original contribution of this comparative study is to widen the description and possible results of federalism with a finer-grained analytical framework for defining the characteristics of decentralization, called the "decision space approach" (Bossert, 1998). We examine the concept of decentralization as a way of fleshing out the concept of federalism with specific attention to the decision space that is defined for the different subnational levels. The concepts are compatible and overlapping. In addition to the constitutional assignment of roles and responsibilities for specific health functions, laws and practice also determine the amount of decision space each level is able to exercise.

Our case study authors used the concept of decision space to assess the degree of choice defined for the subnational levels. Each case developed a "decision space map" which allows us to discuss the general comparative degree of decentralization for decisions about the health sector for the first subnational level and to assess the differences in the decision space for specific functions. In this section we will compare the countries in terms of overall decision space, and in the next section we analyse the different functions separately.

Given all the attention decentralization as a policy has received in recent decades, it is surprising that in many of the federal cases we examined, the decision space for sub-federal levels for most functions is restricted by either constitutional or federal laws to narrow or moderate. Few functions at the subnational level have a wide range of choice. The exceptions are Pakistan and Canada and, to a lesser extent, Brazil.

The cases display a wide variation both in the types of functions that are constitutionally or legally granted to the subnational governments and in the degree of choice over those functions that they are allowed. At one extreme is the Pakistan case, where wide choice has been granted to the provinces for most of the possible functions and where the Ministry of Health was disbanded for over a year and responsibilities for national-level health sector functions were distributed among other ministries. At the other extreme is Germany, where the central government has significant control over many of the functions of the social health insurance schemes and through them the provision of services.

In general we might array the countries from those with the most decentralized to the most centralized health systems (in a manner similar to that used by Requejo (2010) for general political decentralization in plurinational federations) in the following order: Pakistan, Canada, Switzerland, South Africa, Brazil, Mexico, Nigeria, Germany. As this order suggests, among these cases there is no clear argument for decision space to be associated with political (authoritarian or types of democracies) or economic (high, middle, or low income) factors. This order also shows that decentralization in the health sector is likely to be slightly different from the general de facto decentralization that Requejo measured, which for the subset of countries in both studies ranked them as Canada, Switzerland, Germany, Brazil, South Africa, Mexico (see the introduction).

Functions of Decision Space

There are some functions that generally have been reserved to the national level, even in the extremely decentralized case of Pakistan. These include drug quality issues, national immunization campaigns, control of epidemics, negotiation with international donors, and quality control and accreditation. Canada is the exception: these functions are also largely exercised at the provincial level.

While financing decision space varied considerably, all the cases demonstrate that it is important to recognize who holds the purse strings. In Switzerland and Canada, the non-federal levels have significant ability to mobilize their own-source revenues through taxation powers. By contrast, in Germany the health insurance funds are largely dependent on national authority over income and risk definitions as well as for 10 per cent of their funding. In the other countries (Brazil, Pakistan, Mexico, Nigeria, South Africa), the non-federal levels rely on the taxation power of the federation; in these countries the provincial, state, and local authorities are highly reliant on intergovernmental transfers from the federal government. The formality of the assignment formula and the conditionality of the grants have important implications for the decision space of the non-federal levels. Some grants are unconditional and allow states, provinces, or municipalities to make decisions about how much will be allocated to health, while others have significant conditions on subnational choice.

It is also interesting to note that the declining portion of funding from federal sources in Canada (now less than 20 per cent) and Switzerland (only 6 per cent) has led to greater autonomy of the provinces and cantons. In Brazil, despite the decline in central government funding from 75 per cent to 44 per cent, the federal funding remains substantial and supports the dominance of the Unified System. In South Africa, the formula assignment of block grants to the provinces with no conditionality has been relatively low compared to the need and left many provincial health systems with insufficient levels of health funding. In Nigeria, the block grants are unconditional but have resulted in significant differences in health allocations from state to state. State governments and hospital boards in Nigeria can raise fees without federal approval, giving them moderate control over income and expenditures. In South Africa, no fees are allowed for primary care but hospital fees are negotiated between provincial and federal authorities.

Service delivery decision space, including payment mechanisms for facilities, also varies considerably. Germany, Brazil, Mexico, and Nigeria are relatively centralized on the choices of standards and requirements for specific health programs and rules on payments to hospitals. Canada allows some provincial choice based on medically necessary services. By contrast, Switzerland gives wide choice to the cantons. Pakistan allows considerable provincial choice limited mainly by international agreements. Choices over hospital autonomy also varied, with Canada, Switzerland, and Germany allowing wide choice and Mexico allowing state choice, but few states actually use this authority. Brazil, Nigeria, and Pakistan allow a moderate range of choice.

Human resources tend to be one of the most overlooked functional areas, yet it is critical to the ability of subnational governments to administer and regulate health systems. Here, decision space for most subfunctions ranged from wide choice in the Canadian provinces and Swiss cantons to moderate for Mexican, Nigerian, and Brazilian states and German *Länder*. Interestingly, most human resources choices on salaries and civil service rules are still centralized in Pakistan despite the radical devolution of the 18th Amendment. They are also narrow for provinces in South Africa. Nigeria has federal salary rules, but states tend to set their own salaries, resulting in some labour conflicts. Civil service rules are also federally defined in Nigeria. In Germany, federal guidelines on payments allow some variation in the *Länder*. Contracting staff is a cantonal responsibility in Switzerland and a provincial responsibility in Canada and Pakistan. In Mexico, labour agreements limit the provincial authority over contracting staff. Contracting is a federal responsibility in Brazil and South Africa.

Access decisions have two fundamental dimensions. The first is the question of which citizens have access to insurance coverage or services. The second dimension addresses the question of the size of the basket of covered services. Both of these decisions tend to be defined by the constitution or by national-level laws, even in the more decentralized countries of Switzerland and Canada. However, failure to enforce federal rules in Nigeria tends to allow states a moderate range of choice, and even with federal universal access in South Africa, provinces have some choice over priorities. The link to targeting in social welfare programs allows some provincial and cantonal moderate choice in Canada and Switzerland.

Governance rules also varied considerably, with South Africa and Canada having centralized definitions of facility board composition but provincial definition of district offices, while Swiss cantons have moderate choice on boards but wide choice on community participation. Although Mexico allows state decisions about state administrative structure, most follow national models and no facilities have boards. In Brazil the states have authority over boards and district offices. South Africa provinces have moderate choice over community participation, with federal expectation that provinces would encourage community participation. Although there are national guidelines in Nigeria, the lack of enforcement leads to significant variation among local governments. In Germany, the federal government has oversight over national social insurance plans but the states have oversight over state insurers.

Outcomes: Equity of Financing and Health Status

Often a significant issue in decentralization is the effect of local choice on equity of funding, coverage, services, and health outcomes (Bossert, Larrañaga,

Giedion, Arbelaez, & Bowser, 2003). Our cases were not able to assess these impacts in a comparative analysis; however, they do show that some countries have considerable concern about equity and have developed a rationale for federal intervention to achieve greater equity of services and funding (especially Canada and Switzerland), as well as mechanisms of explicit formulas for allocations of resources and standards for service provision and coverage conditions.

Although there are clear differences in health status among the countries in this comparative study, it was also not possible to assess the influence of federalism and decentralization on these outcomes. Health status is influenced by so many different factors, especially economic conditions and educational levels, that the general characteristics of the structure of a health system do not lend themselves to clear causal relationships with health outcomes.

Policy Recommendations

From this review we see that federalism and decentralization have significant variations among countries and that they are complex phenomena which evolve along different countries' specific paths. It is extremely challenging to provide policy recommendations based on lessons from a small group of countries and apply them unmodified to other countries. It is also important to recognize that we do not have clear empirical studies that show the impact of different types of decentralization on health sector outcomes, so we cannot conclude that one type of decentralization produces better performance than another. With these caveats we nonetheless make a few observations that could be useful to policymakers dealing with health system decentralization within federal countries.

First, constitutions seem to play a significant role in defining the range of decision space at all levels. Without clearly specified roles for states, provinces, cantons, and local governments, the range of choice allowed at these subnational levels tends to be assumed by the national level. Therefore, policy advocates for more decentralization might try to introduce clearer subnational responsibilities in either new constitutions or amendments to existing constitutions. In the case of quasi-federations without constitutions that apportion powers and responsibilities between the central state and subnational states, decentralization advocates might consider new laws or amendments to existing laws. Pakistan shows both the opportunity and the risks involved in making these changes.

Second, in more decentralized systems, policies to establish intergovernmental institutions and processes are one way to encourage cooperation and greater policy and program symmetry among the subnational units without absorbing functions into the national level.

Third, policymakers should take into account the political economy of their country and governmental capacities. They should also recognize that greater decision space at subnational levels is likely to be more effective in higher-income democratic countries with more local democratic and administrative capacity than in low-income and less democratic contexts. This capacity constraint in some countries is an important consideration when international organizations are promoting "one-size-fits-all" approaches.

Fourth, while it is not clear that use of the market produces better outcomes, it is likely that policymakers considering policies of decentralization ought to consider the effects of other policies that introduce more market and private-sector choice in the design of their decentralization policies. More use of the market tends to give beneficiaries a greater role in determining the utilization patterns for public services, and the capacities for addressing these new patterns need to be developed at whatever level has more decision space.

Fifth, the current wave of interest in social health insurance makes it important for policymakers considering decentralization policies to also consider the design and implementation of this funding mechanism. If a social health insurance agency is to provide funding directly to health providers, the role of direct public funding through subnational governments will be reduced since they no longer will have the purse strings; however, they may still have influence through coordinating mechanisms and regulations.

Sixth, choices about decision space functions to be assigned to subnational units should consider that in general some functions may be best retained at the federal level: drug quality, immunization campaigns, control of epidemics, negotiation with international donors (in the case of lower-income countries), and quality control and accreditation. Financing choices that encourage greater decision space at local levels are likely to require greater local capacities both to administer those funds and to mobilize additional resources from local taxes and other revenues. Unconditional grants from the federal government are also likely to require strong local capacity to be effective. Due to the heterogeneity of the findings, our study does not provide clear policy guidance on decision space for functions of service delivery, human resources, access rules, and governance.

Finally, more research should be supported by international organizations and development partners to use sophisticated scientific evaluation methodologies to provide clear evidence of the types or degrees of decentralization that are likely to produce better health outcomes. A significant investment in this kind of research could deliver more confident recommendations for policies.

Conclusion

This comparative overview has suggested that the concepts of federalism and decentralization cover a wide variety of actual experience in the different countries. We have identified some relationships between political economy characteristics and elements of federalism and decentralization especially in terms of capacities of health systems, specifically at lower administrative levels. We have also found some interesting policy processes that may be important for future studies, the role of corporatism, and the fragmentation of the health financing systems. For our focus on decision space we find that some functions seem to be retained at the central level even in the most decentralized health systems: drug quality issues, national immunization campaigns, control of epidemics, negotiation with international donors, and quality control and accreditation. Who controls funding also is important in defining the range of choice allowed at lower levels, with greater dependence on central transfers reducing decision space at lower levels. We find, however, for most other functions, variety of decision space does not lead to clear descriptive patterns.

While we make some policy recommendations, these are given with caution and recognized limitations. We unfortunately do not have sufficient scientific evidence to demonstrate which of these varieties has led to improved health system outcomes. The agenda for research now should focus on developing more sophisticated studies of the impact of these different characteristics on the ultimate outcomes we would like to encourage health systems to achieve, especially improved and more equitable health status, reduction of financial risk of illnesses, and general public satisfaction with their systems (see Roberts, Hsiao, Berman, & Reich, 2004).

What this collection demonstrates is that it is important to assess federalism and decentralization in a more fine-grained analysis than the usual more simplistic forms. It is useful to describe both the functions and the range of choice given by the constitutions, other laws and regulations, and actual practice in evidence at the subnational levels to understand the complex relationships embodied in each country's administrative structure. There are quite a variety of forms of decentralization in this optic of "decision space." We have presented eight cases using this analytical framework and have found some generalizations for this limited set of countries. We hope that this approach can be used in more cases to generate a more sophisticated understanding of the widely debated issues of federalism and decentralization.

REFERENCES

Acemoglu, D., & Robinson, J.A. (2012). *Why nations fail: The origins of power, prosperity, and poverty.* New York, NY: Crown Publishing.

Atun, R. (2007). Privatization as a decentralization strategy. In R.B. Saltman, V. Bankauskaite, & K. Vrangbæk (Eds.), *Decentralization in health care* (pp. 246–72). Maidenhead, UK: Open University Press.

Bossert, T.J. (1998). Analyzing the decentralization of health systems in developing countries: Decision space, innovation and performance. *Social Science & Medicine, 47*(10), 1513–27. https://doi.org/10.1016/S0277-9536(98)00234-2

Bossert, T., Larrañaga, O., Giedion, U., Arbelaez, J., & Bowser, D. (2003). Decentralization and equity of resource allocation: Evidence from Colombia and Chile. *Bulletin of the World Health Organization, 81*(2), 95–100.

Costa-Font, J., & Greer, S.L. (Eds.). (2013). *Federalism and decentralization in European health and social care.* Basingstoke, UK: Palgrave Macmillan. https://doi.org/10.1057/9781137291875

Fierlbeck, K., & Palley, H.A. (2015). Conclusion. In K. Fierlbeck & H.A. Palley (Eds.), *Comparative health care federalism* (pp. 213–26). London, UK: Routledge.

Immergut, E.M. (1990). Institutions, veto points, and policy results: A comparative analysis of health care. *Journal of Public Policy, 10*(4), 391–416. https://doi.org/10.1017/S0143814X00006061

Marchildon, G.P. (2009). Postmodern federalism and sub-state nationalism. In A. Ward & L. Ward (Eds.), *The Ashgate research companion to federalism* (pp. 441–55). Farnham, UK: Ashgate.

Nathan, R.P. (1993). The role of the states in American federalism. In C.E. Van Horn (Eds.), *The state of the states* (2nd ed.) (pp. 15–30). Washington, DC: CQ Press.

Requejo, F. (2010). Federalism and democracy: The case of minority nations – a federalist deficit. In M. Burgess & A. Gagnon (Eds.), *Federal democracies* (pp. 275–98). London, UK: Routledge.

Roberts, M., Hsiao, W., Berman, P., & Reich, M. (2004). *Getting health reform right: A guide to improving performance and equity.* Oxford, UK: Oxford University Press.

Saltman, R.B., & Dubois, H.F.W. (2004). The historical and social base of social health insurance systems. In R.B. Saltman, R. Busse, & J. Figueras (Eds.), *Social health insurances in Western Europe* (pp. 21–32). Maidenhead, UK: Open University Press.

Tuohy, C.H. (2009). *Accidental logics: The dynamics of change in the health care arena in the United States, Britain, and Canada.* Oxford, UK: Oxford University Press.

Contributors

Dr Temitope Akintunde is a public health physician with an MPH from Harvard T.H. Chan School of Public Health and a member of McKinsey and Company's Global Health practice in Africa. She was previously a consultant in the World Bank's Health, Nutrition, and Population Global Practice. She has published in the areas of immunization and health systems.

Ogoh Alubo is professor of sociology at the University of Jos, Nigeria. He received his BSc in sociology from Ahmadu Bello University, Zaria, Nigeria, and his MA, MPH, and PhD (sociology) from the University of Missouri–Columbia. He has consulted for Nigerian and international organizations and has published in numerous journals. He is the author of *Medical Professionalism and State Power in Nigeria* (1995) and *Ethnic Conflicts and Citizenship Crises in Central Nigeria* (2011).

Marta Arretche is a full professor of the Department of Political Science at the University of São Paulo and vice provost for research, also at USP. She holds a PhD in social science from the State University of Campinas (UNICAMP). She has been visiting fellow at MIT and the European University Institute. She is editor of the *Brazilian Political Science Review* and director of the Center for Metropolitan Studies. Her research area is institutional and comparative analysis on federalism and social policies.

Leticia Avila-Burgos, MD, PhD, works with the Department of Health Economics at the National Institute of Public Health, Mexico.

Thomas J. Bossert, PhD, is a senior lecturer and the director of the International Health Systems Program of the Harvard T.H. Chan School of Public Health.

: has many years of experience in international health in Latin America and the Caribbean, Africa, Asia, and Central and Eastern Europe. His innovative decision space approach to decentralization has appeared in many prestigious journals and recently in an edited book on decentralization. At Harvard, he teaches courses on health system reform and political economy of health systems. He also teaches in the Harvard/World Bank Flagship Course on Health System Strengthening in Washington and in various countries around the world. Dr Bossert earned his AB from the Woodrow Wilson School at Princeton University and a PhD in political science from the University of Wisconsin, Madison.

Lucero Cahuana Hurtado is an economist, researcher, and professor at the Center for Health Systems Research at the National Institute of Public Health, Mexico. Her research interests focus on the public economy, macroeconomics, health, and the interaction of health systems with economic policies. She is an assistant coordinator of the Masters in Health Systems and manager of "Ideas in Public Health," a space for the dissemination of ideas in public health.

Saniyya Gauhar is a barrister by profession and was editor of the Pakistan-based business magazine *Blue Chip* for four years. A graduate of Sussex University, Saniyya achieved a First Class Honours in contemporary history and later went on to do the Common Professional Examination (CPE) and was called to the Bar in 2000. She is now a freelance writer.

Miguel A. González Block is an associate researcher at the Faculty of Health Sciences, Anahuac University, Mexico. He has been executive director of the Center for Health Systems Research at the National Institute of Public Health of Mexico and was the founding director of Health Policy Research at the National Institute of Public Health. In 1994, he was a founding member of the Center for Economy and Health at the Mexican Health Foundation, where he collaborated with Julio Frenk in the influential study "Economy and Health." From 1999 to 2005, he was the director of the Alliance for Health Policies and Systems Research at the World Health Organization. His publications include several important articles on decentralization in Mexico.

Stefan Greß is associate professor for health services research and health economics in the Department of Health Sciences at the University of Applied Sciences Fulda in Germany. His main areas of research are health policy and health insurance. He has published articles in international peer-reviewed journals on topics such as health services research in primary care, competition and consumer mobility in social health insurance, regulation of pharmaceutical markets, the definition of benefits packages, and the relationship between health insurance and professional autonomy of health care providers.

Stephanie Heinemann is a researcher at the Department for General Practice at the University Medical Center in Göttingen, Germany, and a teacher at the Department of Health Sciences at the University of Applied Sciences Fulda in Germany. Her main areas of research are international comparative health services research, secondary analysis of routine data in primary care, and the analysis of complex interventions.

Gregory P. Marchildon is professor and Ontario Research Chair in Health Policy and System Design at the Institute of Health Policy, Management, and Evaluation, University of Toronto. He is also the founding director of the North American Observatory on Health Systems and Policies. A scholar-practitioner, Marchildon has extensive experience in establishing and working in national and international research and policy networks. A former senior civil servant in the provincial government of Saskatchewan, Marchildon was also the executive director of the Royal Commission on the Future of Health Care in Canada. He has published numerous journal articles and books and is the author of the first and second editions of *Health Systems in Transition: Canada*, a study completed for the European Observatory on Health Systems and Policies. Marchildon is also the Canadian representative on the Health Systems and Policy Monitor network.

Elize Massard da Fonseca is a research fellow at the Center for Business Studies, at the Institute of Education and Research (INSPER) in São Paulo, Brazil. She does research on political economy of public policies, allocation of authority, and regulatory policies, mostly in regard to the health sector and the pharmaceutical industry. Her current research addresses the politics of pharmaceutical regulation in comparative perspective, funded by the São Paulo Research Foundation.

Julia Moorman is public health medicine physician at the School of Public Health, University of the Witwatersrand, Johannesburg, South Africa.

Sania Nishtar is the founder and president of Heartfile. A cardiologist by training, she was Best Graduate of the Khyber Medical College in 1986 and holds a fellowship of the Royal College of Physicians of London and a PhD from King's College London. She combines high-level experiences in government, civil society, and multilateral institutions. As Federal Minister of the Government of Pakistan, she was instrumental in establishing Pakistan's Ministry of Health. Internationally, she is a member of many expert working groups and task forces of WHO and was founding chair of the UN's Independent Accountability Panel for the Global Strategy for Women's, Children's, and Adolescents' Health. She also served as co-chair of the WHO Commission on Ending Childhood Obesity. Dr Nishtar has received the Global Innovation Award for health advocacy work and is a prolific author. In 2017 Dr Nishtar was one of three candidates for director-general of the World Health Organization.

Emanuel Orozco is a research sociologist at the Center for Health Systems Research, National Institute of Public Health, Mexico.

Laetitia C. Rispel is a professor of public health at the University of the Witwatersrand (Wits) in Johannesburg, South Africa. Her research expertise is in public health, specifically health policy and systems research. She is a member of the editorial board of the international *Journal of Public Health Policy* and is the president-elect of the World Federation of Public Health Associations.

Dr Björn Uhlmann received his PhD in political science from the University of Lausanne, where he was also the team leader in a research project on federalism and health governance comparing Switzerland, Germany, and Australia. He has also been a visiting scholar at La Trobe University in Melbourne.

Index